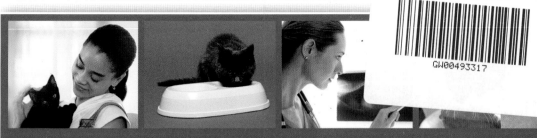

VETERINARY ADVICE FOR

Cat owners

Oesophagus Lungs Kidneys

Heart

Bladder

Liver Stomach Spleen

A COMPLETE HOME REFERENCE GUIDE

Bronchi

Bronchiolos

Lung Alveolus

Trevor Turner, BVet Med, MRCVS
and Jean Turner

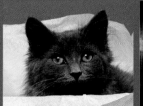
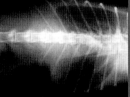
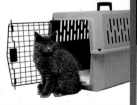
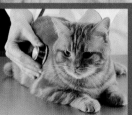

ACKNOWLEDGEMENTS

The publishers would like to acknowledge the following for help with photography: Jean and Trevor Turner, and Angela Tyrrell.

page 11 © istockphoto.com/Vladimir Suponev.

Cover photography: **Main Cover Image:** © www.comstock.com.

Top Sequence, left-right: © www.comstock.com; © istockphoto.com/Brian McEntire;
© www.comstock.com; © www.comstock.com.

Bottom sequence: © www.comstock.com; © istockphoto.com/Chiya Li;
© www.comstock.com; © www.comstock.com.

First published in 2010 by The Pet Book Publishing Company Limited
PO Box 8, Lydney, Gloucestershire GL15 6YD

© 2010 Pet Book Publishing Company Limited.

ISBN
978-1-906305-12-3
1-906305-12-9

Printed and bound in Singapore.

CONTENTS

INTRODUCTION

The estimated figures vary according to the source, but it is agreed that cats have outstripped dogs as the most popular pets in Britain and the USA. It is known that at least 8 million homes in Britain have accepted the responsibility of looking after a cat. In the US, there is an amazing 77 million owned cats – 34 per cent of all US households own at least one cat.

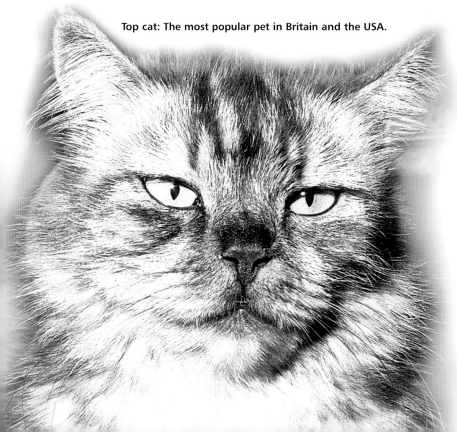

Top cat: The most popular pet in Britain and the USA.

Over the last decade, it has come to be realised that cats are much less labour intensive to own than dogs, and this fits in with the increased pace of modern life.

Care still has to be taken with selection. For example, Persians and other longhaired cats need careful daily grooming, which is very time consuming. However, cats, unlike dogs, do not need to be taken out for exercise on a daily basis – although this does not mean that they do not need regular exercise. The Fat Cat syndrome is recognised by veterinarians as a term applying not only to certain entrepreneurs but as a recognised medical problem with our feline friends.

However, an exercise regime for portly cats is still less demanding than that for their canine counterparts. There is no five-mile daily slog in all weathers! Exercise from a gleam of light, be it a hand mirror or a pen torch is all that is required. Most of our feline friends will instinctively want to kill that spot of light – armchair exercise indeed!

PERFECT PETS

Feline popularity has brought its own problems. Rescue homes, cat sanctuaries and the "lady down the road who takes in cats" have, during the last few years, become overwhelmed with unwanted cats of all descriptions. These include elderly homeless moggies moved from their familiar home territory and truly lost, pedigree Persians whose owners cannot cope with the responsibilities of coat care, and the victims of a breakdown in owner relationships.

Cats may be the most popular pets but they do not enjoy quite so much consideration for their future as their canine counterparts. This, in part, may be due to their independence, which is certainly an asset to cat keeping in today's society. Novice owners are often misled into thinking that because of the cat's inherent independence, it is well able to look after itself. Some cats end up in rescue solely because they have been translocated to a new abode, not become sufficiently bonded with it, and then use their independence to try to regain their old haunts. Amazingly some do – sometimes walking tremendous distances. This, however, is the exception rather than the rule. Many depend on benevolent neighbours – some become almost nomadic and add to the total statistics without being really owned by anyone. Others get taken into rescue, but many are injured in road traffic accidents and so become statistics of a different kind.

The take-home message is loud and clear: share your home with a cat by all means, but be responsible. Accept that the commitment is for the life of the cat, which is statistically longer than that of a dog.

HOW DO YOU CHOOSE A CAT?

- Do you want a non-pedigree (moggie) or a pedigree kitten?
- Do you want a kitten, or would you prefer to give a home to a full-grown mature cat? Most cat homes are more than relieved when they get enquiries regarding adult cats.

They are all available, pedigree and non-pedigree alike! Pedigree cats and kittens can be obtained through breed rescue organisations, and from breeders directly. Today, on the web, there are many cat-specific sites, and a couple of hours' surfing will reveal an immense choice.

Start with the following website – www.thecatgroup.org.uk –

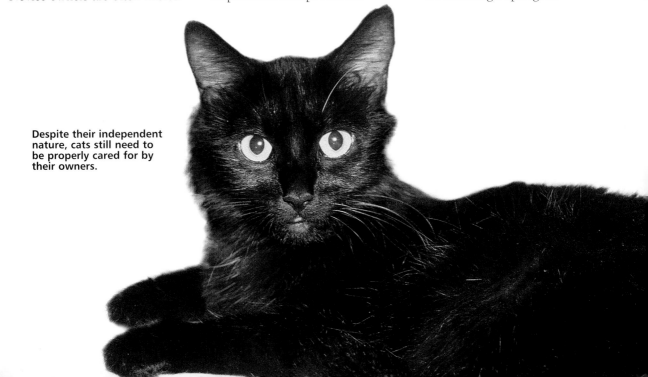

Despite their independent nature, cats still need to be properly cared for by their owners.

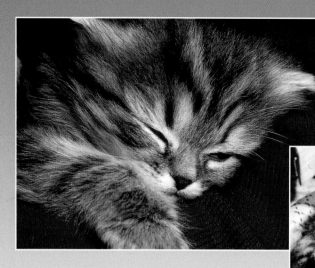

Is your heart set on finding a kitten?

Or do you want to rehome an adult cat?

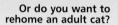

where there is a page explaining how to go about finding a cat. This covers moggies and pedigrees, kittens and adults. There is also the Feline Advisory Bureau, www.fabcats.org.uk, with an information sheet, Choosing a Pedigree Kitten:

What to Expect.

There are also many rescue organisations, which include the RSPCA, www.rspca.org.uk, Cats Protection, www.cats.org.uk, the Blue Cross, www.bluecross.org.uk, as well as Battersea Dogs and Cats Home, www.dogshome.org.uk

and Wood Green Animal Shelters, www.woodgreen.org.uk

If you would like to restrict your search to your local area, try your veterinary surgeon for local breeders. Yellow Pages list the addresses of local rescue organisations.

PART I

CARING FOR YOUR CAT

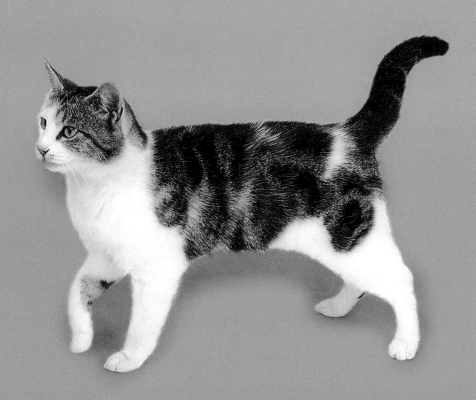

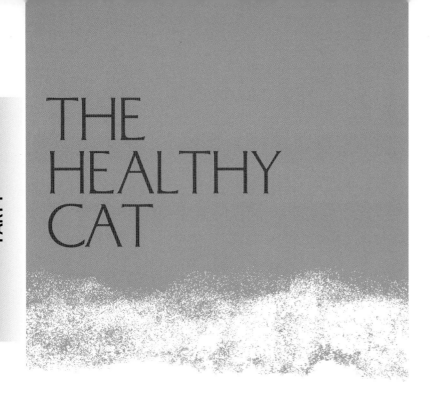

THE HEALTHY CAT

Chapter 1

P ick up any modern cat care manual and you will find many words written on the subject of feline health, but very few describing the healthy cat. Those that do, invariably list common signs of ill health, leaving you to deduce the signs of health.

Many times throughout this book I mention that cats will often conceal their true feelings. When ill, the cat will endeavour to behave normally for as long as possible, thus making it difficult to spot if anything is wrong. Owners, knowing their cat's habits, are often in a much better position than even their vet, to

be able to differentiate when the cat is out of sorts. Many caring owners will tell stories of having taken their cat to the vet, who couldn't find anything wrong, only to have a very sick cat a few days later. Clearly they spotted the problem before the vet did!

This is solely due to the intuitive ability of an observant owner to detect very subtle changes in habits, behaviour or personality of the cat. It is really all about getting to know your cat's character, and noticing particular foibles that alert you to the first signs of illness or injury – something denied initially to even the most observant vet.

SIGNS OF HEALTH

COAT
With kittens and adult cats, the coat is a good indicator of health. It reflects a good diet and general

The bright, alert expression of the eyes, which is synonymous with good health.

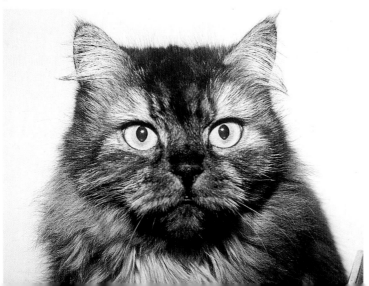

SIGNS OF GOOD HEALTH

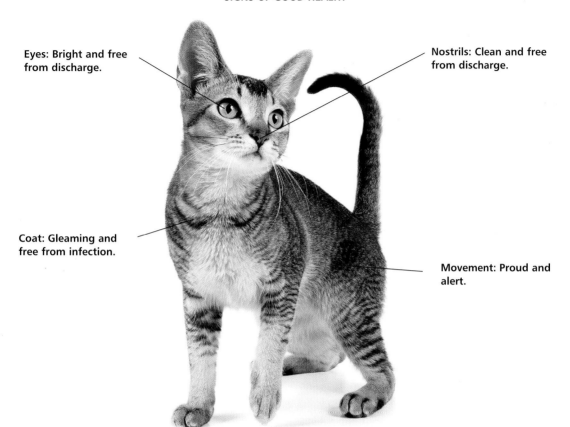

Eyes: Bright and free from discharge.

Nostrils: Clean and free from discharge.

Coat: Gleaming and free from infection.

Movement: Proud and alert.

condition. It should be gleaming and free from scurf or dandruff, no matter whether the cat is short or longhaired. Gently parting the hair and looking at the skin will give an indication of any fleas or other ectoparasites. Sores, pimples and bare patches are also revealed.

EYES
Eyes are also considered the barometer of health. They should be bright with an alert expression. There should be no discharge, redness or undue blinking.

NOSTRILS
There should be no discharge from the nostrils. Both should be clean.

MOVEMENT
The cat should move with a proudly carried tail and an alert expression, exuding the inborn confidence of the supreme, superb predator.

POSITIVE INDICATORS
Having gained an overall impression of the state of the cat, how do you then confirm your impression of health? Here are a

few tips that make the task easier.

HEARING
Cats are renowned for their sense of hearing; therefore, they should be alert to any sudden noise. If this is ignored, and particularly if the cat is white-coloured, deafness should be suspected since this can often be congenital deafness linked to a white coat colour.

BREATHING
This should be regular and silent. Signs of noisy breathing are often an indication of respiratory

PART I

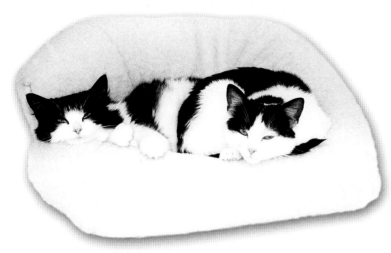

A healthy cat will have a good appetite and be calm and contented in the home environment.

problems. The respiratory rate in the cat is normally about 20-30 breaths per minute. It is usually barely perceptible, and not in any way laboured.

THIRD EYELID

Cats do not normally show their haws, i.e. the third eyelid or nictitating membrane. It usually concealed at the inner corners (nasal edge) of the eye. If it is prominent, it is often a sign of illness.

EARS

Check the ears. They should be clean with no evidence of excess wax or odour. Gently stroke the face around the ears and the ear itself. Most cats enjoy this; scratching or rubbing indicates problems with the ear canals, usually due to mites.

MOUTH

If possible, try to examine the mouth. Place one hand over the upper jaw and use a finger nail

on the lower incisors. This usually results in the cat opening the mouth, giving you enough time to make sure that the gums are a healthy pink colour. The teeth should be white and clean, with only minimal evidence of tartar (calculus) or bad breath, depending on age.

BODY

Run your hands over the body and make sure there are no lumps, bumps or sore places. Run your hand down to the tip of the tail to make sure it is straight and free from deformity. While at the rear end it is advisable to check the anus and genitals, which should be clean and free from any sign of diarrhoea or discharge.

With your own cat you can check further by examining the faeces, which should be firm although some cats will periodically have loose stools without showing any signs of ill health.

VOMITING

Healthy cats will vomit occasionally, bringing up fur balls. This is a natural defence mechanism and is not a cause for concern, provided it does not happen too often. Some cats will vomit merely because they have eaten too much too rapidly, or occasionally when an unpalatable insect or creature has been caught and consumed.

It is normal for healthy cats to chew vegetation, particularly grass. Sometimes they chew the wrong type of vegetation and this will cause them to vomit. However, this should not be persistent.

NORMAL TEMPERATURE

The normal rectal temperature is around 38-38.5 degrees Centigrade (100.5-101.5 Fahrenheit). Unless you have experience, it is not easy to accurately take a cat's temperature by putting a thermometer up the bottom. Don't worry – a reasonable indication that the cat has a raised temperature is if the ears feel hot to a gentle touch.

WHEN TO CALL THE VET

This is not as simple as it seems, since, as mentioned previously, if you are acting on a hunch, the vet may not be able to find anything amiss, despite careful clinical examination. It is therefore always worth making a written record (dated and timed) of any signs that are abnormal, as well as a note of general changes in behaviour, attitude etc.

SIGNS AND SYMPTOMS

These are frequently referred to in respect of health and disease.

- **Signs:** These present objective evidence that something is wrong. They are considered to be easily noticed, even by a casual observer, e.g. diarrhoea, sneezing, lack of appetite.
- **Symptoms:** These are changes in sensation and bodily function that can only be experienced by the subject, e.g. sudden backache, indigestion, etc.

Strictly speaking, symptoms should only be used in relation to human problems since cats cannot tell us how they are feeling. Throughout this book, I have tried to refer solely to signs of disease – although the terms are very often used synonymously today.

You will note that this section is headed – When To Call The Vet – not When To Go To The Vet. It is always a good rule to take advice earlier rather than later, and at least alert the practice of a possible problem. Do not be afraid to telephone.

EMERGENCIES

There is obviously little doubt regarding seeking professional

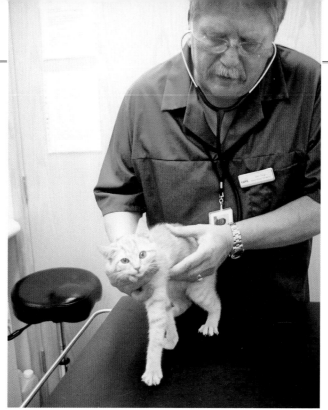

All cats should have a regular check-up with the vet.

advice in emergency situations if the cat is:

- Shocked or haemorrhaging
- Obviously injured
- Appears partially or completely unconscious
- Is falling about with uncoordinated movements

The difficulty is with situations where the cat is vomiting or has diarrhoea. Cats do vomit and will pass loose stools on occasions but if this is repetitive, veterinary advice is needed. Similarly, cats will chase and catch stinging insects and sometimes get bitten or stung and suffer anaphylaxis – an allergic reaction involving acute swelling of the injured part. If this should happen to be the mouth or the throat through swallowing a bee, the results can

be very serious and urgent veterinary attention is required.

If the cat appears to be unproductively straining either to pass urine or faeces, this is another cause for concern since this can be due to constipation or a serious urinary blockage.

More difficult are insidious changes involving loss of weight. Few of us regularly weigh our cats, and sometimes weight loss can be so gradual that it is not noticed at first. If you have any worries – even if the cat appears to be well in every other way – a check-up with the vet is worthwhile.

REGULAR CHECK-UPS

As a result of the vaccination debate, one point to emerge has been the emphasis on the need for regular, at least annual, check-ups, even if booster vaccinations are not being given.

With our cats, just as with us, increasing age means regular check-ups are all the more important. In the case of the cat, dental plus heart and respiratory problems can often be picked up and successfully stabilised, if not cured, if caught in time. Similarly, the regular check-up will also reveal the presence of lumps and bumps, which can be investigated before it is too late.

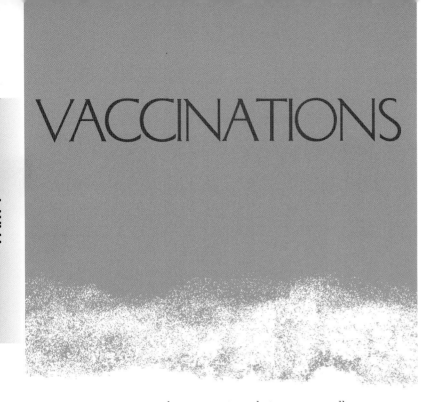

VACCINATIONS

Chapter 2

Vaccinations and inoculations – is there any difference? For most owners, and vets for that matter, there is very little difference. The terms are often used synony-mously. Strictly speaking, inoculations are usually associated with injections, e.g. "How much is a feline enteritis inoculation?" or "I'm going to get his flu jabs done." Implicit in the remarks is the fact that the procedure will involve an injection.

Vaccination tends to have a broader meaning. For example, some vaccines can be administered in the form of nasal drops, e.g. feline Bordetella vaccine. Today, irrespective of the method by which the cat is protected, we still talk about a vaccination programme – even though the cat may have been injected against various diseases.

VACCINATION CONTROVERSY

Feline vaccination programmes are presently just as contentious as those for our children. Arguments centre on how many different components should be incorporated into any one vaccine, how often should they be repeated, i.e. boosted, and does the combination of these components overload the immune system?

Having been around since before the advent of widespread

If you are concerned about vaccinations, discuss the matter with your vet.

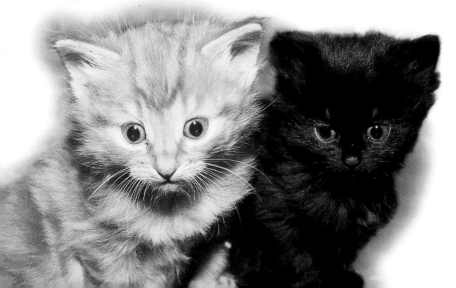

feline vaccination, it is my view that these arguments and discussions have only really arisen due to the overall efficacy of these vaccines in the first place. Killer diseases, e.g. feline enteritis and cat flu, have both been largely controlled if not eradicated in the pet cat population. I am convinced that this is due to the widespread use of safe, effective vaccines.

Once vaccination has minimised the risk of disease, any untoward reaction as a result of the vaccine itself obviously assumes major importance. In over 40 years of very intensive feline practice, I have personally experienced very few reactions – although I have used a wide variety of feline vaccines. Consequently, I am convinced that the benefits of vaccination far outweigh the risks.

However, I can appreciate the viewpoint of those who have had a perfectly healthy animal vaccinated and had a reaction as a result. Nonetheless, this is a very rare occurrence. If you are concerned about this issue, it is important that you discuss it with your vet.

VACCINATION REACTIONS

We know that reactions are more likely to occur with repeat vaccinations, i.e. booster jabs, and today the move is towards individual assessment of the risks and benefits for each cat rather than an overall booster programme. Some components of multivalent (combined) vaccines can now be boosted separately if

preferred. However, this is likely to cost more, and I am rather ambivalent regarding the cat's welfare, since more injections are necessary.

From the cat's point of view, it is surely less stressful to use multivalent vaccines rather than have to return to the vet several times in order to receive separate injections of the individual components?

It must be remembered that no vaccine can carry 100 per cent guarantee of either safety or efficacy. In both the UK and North America, any vaccine – no matter whether to protect against one disease (monovalent) or against a clutch of diseases (multivalent) – has to satisfy the licensing authorities regarding safety and efficacy before a manufacturer's licence will be granted. Very occasionally the

vaccine does not come up to expectations. However, in general, feline vaccines are very effective.

In the UK, in addition to rigorous testing procedures for efficacy and safety, there is also an obligation to report any suspected adverse reactions to the manufacturer. As a result, a much more reliable picture of vaccine-induced reactions is emerging, and it does appear that genuine vaccine reactions are very low. Thus, the risks are very low compared with the risks to the cat if a decision is made not to vaccinate at all.

CORE VACCINES

These are those for which routine vaccination is recommended for all cats based upon the seriousness of the disease, difficulty of treating it or its

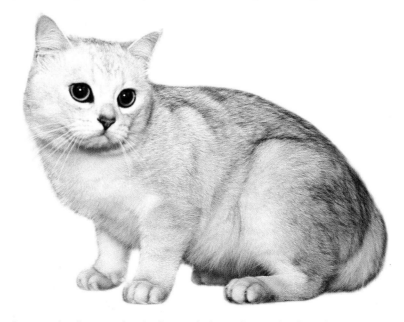

Core vaccinations need to be boosted, depending on local conditions.

PART I

widespread prevalence.
In Britain the core vaccines are generally recognised as:

- Panleucopaenia (FPV) also known as feline infectious enteritis (FIE)
- Flu viruses, i.e. feline herpes virus (FHV) also known as feline viral rhinotracleitis virus (FVR) and feline calicivirus (FCV.)
- In countries where rabies is endemic, e.g. parts of the United States, to this list should be added rabies.

Core vaccines should be boosted according to manufacturers' recommendations, usually at about fifteen months of age and then as recommended according to local conditions and the cat's lifestyle, etc.

NON-CORE VACCINES
These are needed when there is a genuine increased risk:

- Feline immunodeficiency virus (FIV)
- Feline leukaemia virus (FeLV)

- Feline chlamydophila vaccine
- Feline coronovirus (FCoV) is available in some areas in order to offer protection against feline infectious peritonitis (FIP).
- Feline ringworm vaccines are available in the US, although not at present licensed in Britain.

PEDIGREE KITTENS
The regulating bodies for pedigree cats (GCCF in the UK) advise that kittens should not go to new homes until they are over 13 weeks old. One of the reasons for this is that primary vaccination can be completed, and the kitten can have built up some protection, before being exposed to the stress and different germs of its new home. This is particularly important if there are already other resident cats, even though they may be fully inoculated. This is because, in some cases, cats may be protected by vaccination from the signs of the disease, yet still carry, and actually shed, the causal organisms to which any newcomer – particularly a kitten – could be susceptible.

It should be remembered that with some diseases vaccination protects against the disease, but not against actual infection. A healthy cat may be shedding virus that a susceptible kitten or cat could pick up.

NON-PEDIGREE KITTENS
If the intended new kitten is not a pedigree, and not fully inoculated when you get it, contact your veterinary surgeon without delay to discuss the best vaccination strategy. This will depend not only on the age, breed or type and condition of the kitten, but also the problems of local feline disease. It also depends on the source of the kitten, e.g. private home, rescue centre, etc.

Generally, it is advised that any kitten receives the primary course of core vaccines. These usually cover feline enteritis (panleucopaenia [FPV]), also known in the UK as feline infectious enteritis (FIE), and also the main cat flu viruses, which are calicivirus (FCV) and feline viral rhinotracheitis virus (FVR) – which, to make matters complicated, is also known as feline herpes virus (FHV).

Protection for a kitten under 12 weeks usually involves two injections about 2-3 weeks apart. Ideally, the second injection of vaccine should be put in when the kitten is 10-12 weeks old, depending on manufacturers' recommendations. It then takes about a week to 10 days for the kitten to develop a workable immunity (see Chapter 19).

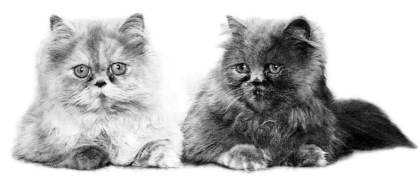

Pedigree kittens, like these blue-cream and blue Persians, should not go to new homes until they are 13 weeks of age.

DO CAT VACCINES CAUSE CANCER?

Very occasionally feline vaccines will cause a reaction. Recently, it has come to light that an extremely low percentage of cats react to some inoculations especially feline leukaemia and rabies. Of these, a further small percentage go on to develop cancerous lumps at the injection site. The situation has been carefully scrutinised by the licensing authorities in Britain and the US. It is acknowledged that this risk does occur, but is very small compared with the risk of the cat getting the disease that the vaccine is aimed to protect against. However, it is worthwhile discussing this with your vet at the time of inoculation. You can then make an informed decision depending upon the circumstances.

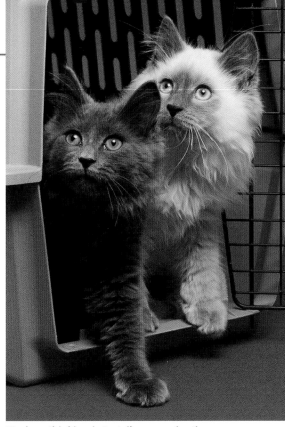

Modern thinking is to tailor a vaccination programme to the individual cat.

We cannot start primary vaccinations until the kitten is about eight weeks of age because the circulating antibodies acquired from the queen will combine with the vaccine antigen, and destroy it, before it has time to stimulate the kitten to produce its own antibodies.

Many rescue centres today follow the recommendations of GCCF and ensure that kittens only go to suitable new homes after they have been fully vaccinated and built up some immunity, i.e. at about 12-13 weeks of age.

KITTENS FROM PRIVATE HOMES

These are often acquired much earlier than three months of age and if the kitten does appear very young, again veterinary advice is essential. Feline enteritis and cat flu (core vaccines) are always needed plus, sometimes, other protection, e.g. feline leukaemia. This is normally regarded as non-core, but if the kitten is destined to go out a lot and meet semi-feral cats, it is well worthwhile. Similarly, chlamydophila vaccine (non-core) is worthwhile if the kitten is coming into a household with a lot of other cats.

These are examples of how the thinking regarding feline vaccination has changed. No longer is it recommended that every cat should have a primary vaccination against every inoculable disease followed by regular, usually annual, boosters.

Today the strategy is very much to tailor vaccinations to the individual cat, ensuring that a primary course of core vaccines is administered and boosted at about 15 months of age. Following boosters will then depend very much on local conditions, i.e. does the cat go out a lot, or is it a house cat? Your vet is the best person to advise.

Non-core vaccines are administered according to local need, e.g. if the cat is frequently boarded, regular flu boosters will be required and, in some cases, Bordetella also. If the cat goes out a lot and is likely to meet with other cats, vaccination against feline leukaemia virus (non-core) is worthwhile maintaining throughout the cat's life.

PARASITES

A parasite is defined as any organism that lives on or within another living organism (the host) from which it obtains some advantage. Parasites can be broadly divided into **ectoparasites,** which live and feed on the outside of the animal, such as fleas, lice, mites etc., and **endoparasites,** which live within the body, e.g. adult tapeworms and roundworms. These, although living in the intestine, lay eggs that are passed out in the faeces and can infect other cats.

Feline ectoparasites may spend all their life cycle on the cat (e.g. lice and mange mites), or use the cat only to obtain nourishment, usually blood, (e.g. fleas and ticks). Sometimes, there is not direct transmission. The eggs or larvae may have to infect an intermediate host, e.g. mice, which in turn have to be eaten by the cat in order to complete the life cycle.

ECTOPARASITES

The main ectoparasites of the cat are fleas, lice, ticks, ear mites, fur mites, harvest mites, notoedric mange, and ringworm (see page 43, Skin).

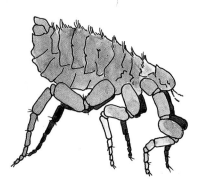

Adult flea – *Ctenocephalides felis.*

FLEAS

Fleas are not particularly host specific. This is the reason why we sometimes get bitten as a result of fleas on our pets. Nevertheless, not surprisingly, the cat flea, *Ctenocephalides felis* (approximately 2.5 mm), is the most common flea found on cats. Outdoor cats that roam frequently can also host hedgehog fleas and rabbit fleas if living in suburban or rural areas.

The life cycle of the flea varies from about three weeks up to two years depending on environmental and climatic conditions. Temperature and humidity are particularly important.

It is only adult fleas that normally live on the cat. They feed on the cat's blood since this is necessary for the completion of their life cycle. Then they may leave the cat to lay eggs in the environment, although sometimes these are laid in the cat's fur and subsequently drop off to hatch in the environment. Historically, flea-induced skin problems were always seasonal and worse in late summer and early autumn, when flea activity is at its peak. Today, with widespread use of central heating, feline flea-induced problems tend to observe no seasonal constraints. However, with widespread use of effective flea control agents on both cat and environment, these problems have declined dramatically during the last decade.

LICE

Lice are more host-specific than fleas although they will occasionally find other hosts, including us. Lice are easier to control since they live and breed on the cat. They lay eggs that are sticky (nits), which attach to the hairs. Lice tend to infect longer-haired cats, probably for this reason!

Lice are approximately the same size as fleas. The only louse of any importance in the cat is the biting louse *Felicola subrostratis*. It has a worldwide distribution, and occasionally causes health problems, particularly with poorly reared or feral cats.

TICKS

Many animals, including man, can be infested with ticks. They have long been recognised as ectoparasites of the cat, particularly in country areas where sheep ticks readily infest cats in order to obtain a blood meal. Suburban cats are more commonly infested with hedgehog ticks.

There are many varieties of ticks, which are not too host specific. They are larger than fleas measuring 5-10 mm in length. The majority that affect cats are grey, bean-shaped parasites. Worried owners will often present cats to their vet thinking they have developed a cyst or growth since the ticks, with their hard bodies, do not move on the cat, having buried their mouth parts beneath the skin in order to feed on the feline blood. They then fall from the cat and complete their lifecycle on the ground, finally crawling up vegetation to await a passing host in order to repeat the cycle. This may take several days.

In some parts of the world, including North America, feline tick infestation is relatively common. Several serious diseases can be transmitted by ticks, some of which are zoonotic (communicable to us). This is now important in the UK with the introduction of PETS, the Pet Travel Scheme, which allows cats (and dogs) to enter and re-enter the UK from approved countries without undergoing quarantine, provided they fulfil the strict entry regulations. Therefore, 'foreign' ticks carrying these diseases could enter Britain on cats (or dogs) coming in under PETS.

In consequence, dogs and cats entering Britain under PETS have

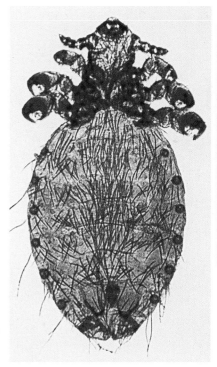

Adult louse (magnified).

to receive appropriate tick (and tapeworm) treatment between 24 - 48 hours before entry.

MITES

Various types of mites cause problems for the cat. Bearing in mind that the external ear is part of the skin, ear mites are the most common type of mite found on the cat. They are highly contagious and can pass from cats to dogs and vice versa. In some cases, they can cause intense irritation.

- **Eat mites:** Ear mites (*Otodectes cyanotis*) are just visible to the naked eye (0.4 mm long). In very heavy infestations, the mites can be found on the hair surrounding the ear and also the root of the tail, since cats often sleep with their head resting around that area.

- **Cheyletiella (fur) mites:** Cheyletiellosis – to use the proper name – is often called 'walking dandruff', which is appropriate. These mites are tiny, only just visible to the naked eye (0.4 mm). They literally look like tiny bits of scale or dandruff moving between the hairs. They live within the scales and debris on the skin surface, which, in turn, increases in proportion to the amount of infestation. Different species infest different animals, but usually they are not host-specific. Consequently, species found on dogs and rabbits will be equally at home on the cat.
- **Mange mites:** Scabies or mange does occur in cats, but it is extremely rare. If it does occur, it is usually due to a mite called *Notoedres cati* and not *Sarcoptes scabii,* which is the common cause in dogs. On rare occasions *Sarcoptes scabii* has been found on cats, but usually when living with mangy dogs!
- **Harvest mites:** Another mite that causes problems in certain parts of the UK and North America is the so-called harvest mite (berry bug, U.S), *Trombicula (Neotrombicula) autumnalis.* The larval mite targets outdoor cats (as well as humans and other animals), particularly those living in

rural areas with chalky soil. It occurs mainly in late summer. The adult mite lives in rotting vegetation and is not parasitic, whereas the larval (immature) form infests the feet, head and the ears of the host cat. These larval mites are tiny but can just be seen by the naked eye, (approximately 0.2 mm). They appear as bright orange dots on the skin.

RINGWORM
Ringworm is often included in any discussion on ectoparasites but is strictly an infection. It is an important condition in the cat. It is not caused by a worm but a fungus. The lesions are seldom circular in the cat – although it can happen! This is fully discussed in the chapter on Skin Problems, see page 43.

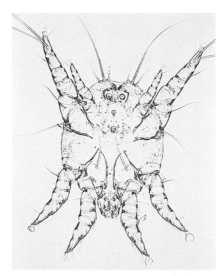

Adult Otodectic mite (magnified)
Otodectes cyanotis.

MAGGOTS
Few of us think of maggots as ectoparasites, but myiasis (fly strike) is not uncommon in run-down, sick outdoor cats in summer time, particularly if their coats become contaminated with urine, faeces or other discharges. Maggots, the larvae of the blowfly, burrow under the skin-producing enzymes that digest the tissue and cause extensive subcutaneous ulceration. When the ambient temperature is high, the maggots can hatch within hours of the eggs being laid.

This requires extensive clipping and removal of all the maggots and cleansing, either with saline (1 teaspoonful of salt to a pint of water) or an appropriately diluted disinfectant safe for use with cats.

ENDOPARASITES
Endoparasites are those that live inside the cat. The most well known are worms which live in the cat's intestines. They are broadly of two types: nematodes (or roundworms) and cestodes (or tapeworms). There are also other endoparasites, although less common, which can cause problems.

LUNGWORM
The lungworm *Aerostrongylus abstrusus* is recognised as a common endoparasite of the respiratory system and has a worldwide distribution. It has been estimated that over a quarter of all domestic cats harbour the parasite. In many

ways it could be considered as the perfect parasite since, very seldom, is it a cause of problems for the cat. This usually only occurs in cats that have other health problems, for example are immunologically incompetent due to FIV, FeLV etc.

The worms are tiny and look like pieces of black thread. Eggs are laid in the lungs and hatch into first-stage larvae, which make their way up the air passages to the pharynx. From here, they are either swallowed or passed to the outside. If swallowed, they complete their life cycle by being carried from the bowel in the bloodstream back to the lungs, where they mature. If the larvae leave the cat, they have to be eaten by an intermediate host. These are usually slugs and snails. If these are eaten by birds, rats or mice, the larvae find their way back to the cat as the result of instinctive feline hunting habits.

ROUNDWORMS (NEMATODES)

Roundworms are aptly named, as they are round-shaped worms measuring 10-15 cm (4-6 in) in length and live in the small intestine. Male worms (10 cm) are smaller than females (15 cm).

There are two types of roundworm found in the cat: *Toxocara cati* and *Toxascaris leonina*. *Toxocara* is by far the more common and has a much more complicated life cycle. Some *Toxocara* larvae actually encyst within the body tissues. In the female cat, some of these only

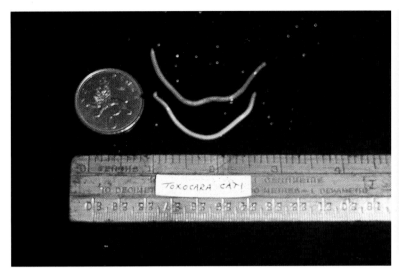

Roundworm – *Toxocara cati*.

then complete their life cycle when stimulated by the hormones secreted during pregnancy. These stimulate the larvae to cross the placental barrier in the bloodstream to become adult in the kitten's bowel. Kittens can then be shedding eggs from the mature worms as early as 11 days after birth.

TAPEWORMS (CESTODES)

Tapeworms consist of a series of flattened segments, each of which contains male and female organs. The segments are continually produced just behind the 'head' (scolex) of the worm, which is embedded in the wall of the cat's small intestine. The segments mature and ultimately break off the rear end of worm and are passed out in the faeces. They are capable of movement when passed, and look like grains of rice or cucumber seeds.

Unlike roundworms, an intermediate host is necessary for completion of the life cycle and this varies according to the type of tapeworm:

- *Dipylidium caninum* is the most common tapeworm infecting cats and the intermediate host is usually a flea or a louse.
- *Taenia taeniaformis* is also very common in the UK and the US and this tapeworm utilises rodents, primarily rats and mice, as intermediate hosts. The life cycle is completed in the cat when it consumes the intermediate host.
- *Echinococcus multilocularis* is the species for which specific anti-tapeworm treatment is necessary for cats entering Britain under the PETS scheme (as mentioned above). This tapeworm is relatively rare in the cat, but there is a risk since humans can act as hosts.

Feline tapeworms are found in many parts of the world including the UK and North America. Most species grow to about 25-30 cm (10-12 in) before mature segments are shed. *Echinococcus* species are the exception. They are very small, barely reaching half a centimetre, less than a quarter of an inch.

HOOKWORMS

Ancylostoma species are prevalent in warm climates, including southern parts of the USA, but are not generally found in Britain.

SIGNS OF WORM INFESTATION

Roundworms and tapeworms seldom cause significant signs in otherwise healthy cats. Wormy kittens often appear small and under-nourished, and can have a distended abdomen (pot belly). Tapeworm segments can frequently be seen moving out of the anus, and will occasionally cause irritation, resulting in the kitten dragging its bottom along the ground (scooting).

Worm treatments both for tapeworm and roundworm are readily available without a

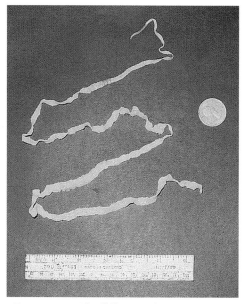

Tapeworm – *Dipylidium caninum.*

prescription from retail outlets. However, it is advisable to consult your vet since accurate diagnosis is worthwhile since some of these worms can be transmitted to humans, particularly children.

Effective, safe preparations are available on prescription that will eradicate both roundworms and tapeworms with a single dose.

OTHER ENDOPARASITES

TOXOPLASMA GONDII

This is a microscopic protozoan, single-celled parasite, often regarded as a feline infection rather than a feline parasite. It is significant since it can be transmitted to us, via the cat's faeces, and cause abortion in pregnant women. However, the infective form takes 2-4 days to develop after the oocysts (eggs) have been voided; therefore there is little danger of infection, provided litter trays are cleaned on a daily basis.

Toxoplasma is usually symptomless, unless the cat is immunosuppressed (e.g. has FIV or FeLV infection), then recurrent diarrhoea sometimes with ocular and nervous signs can occur.

GIARDIASIS

Giardia is another microscopic organism that either can be classified as a parasite or an infection. *Giardia* usually causes intermittent diarrhoea in cats. This is usually self-limiting. However, drugs are available on prescription, which are very effective. The main importance lies in the fact it can cause similar signs with us, but whether it is truly zoonotic has not to date been fully established.

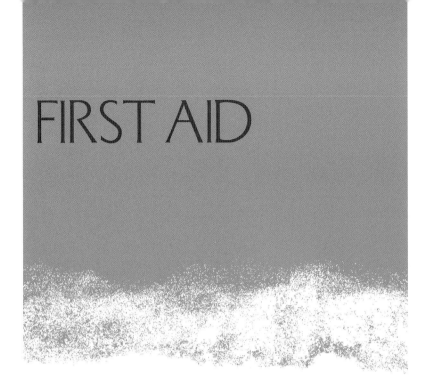

FIRST AID

First aid is the initial treatment given in any emergency, irrespective of its cause. It is important since it can frequently be life-saving. It is essential to get the priorities in order.

WHAT ARE THE PRIORITIES?
- Keep calm and do not panic.
- Try to contact your own veterinary surgeon, but always ensure veterinary help is available. Contacting a practice will often result in specific first-aid advice being given appropriate for the problem.
- If the cat is injured, restrain him if possible. A cardboard box, with a cover to prevent escape, will do if a cat container is not available. Make a few holes for ventilation.
- If the cat is clearly fading or unconscious, try to conserve body heat. Place a towel or

piece of clothing over the entire cat in the box.
- Take the cat to the vet ASAP. Drive carefully and observe speed limits.

WHAT ARE THE AIMS OF FIRST AID?
1. To prevent further injury.
2. To stabilise the cat prior to receiving professional attention.
3. To alleviate pain and suffering if possible.
4. To aid recovery.

THE ABC OF FIRST AID

A: AIRWAY
Make sure the airway is clear. Examine the mouth, opening the jaws with gloved hands, or with the aid of a pen or the handle of a teaspoon wrapped in a handkerchief or tissue.

Remember that even the friendliest cat can be

unpredictable if in pain. Clear any vomit, saliva or blood clots from the mouth with the same makeshift instrument.

B: BREATHING
Check if the cat is breathing. If not, an effective means of artificial respiration is to gently hold the chest just behind the front legs and press and relax, once every couple of seconds.

C: CARDIAC FUNCTION
Is the heart beating? Try to feel a heart beat with your thumb and forefinger, just behind the elbows. If no heart beat is felt, use the thumb and forefinger to massage the chest, at the same time using compression to assist breathing, as **B** above.

FIRST-AID EQUIPMENT
A secure top-opening cat carrier is an essential piece of equipment. If not available, you

have to make do, but try to ensure the cat is as secure as possible. Unconscious cats can suddenly regain consciousness en route to the vet and fight with tooth and claw.

FIRST-AID KIT

Human first-aid kits are readily available, but not all the contents are suitable for feline emergencies. Essential contents of a feline first-aid kit include:

- Blunt-ended scissors for cutting bandages, plasters, etc
- Eyebrow or similar flat-ended tweezers for removing grass seeds, etc
- Assorted bandages and dressings, 2.5 cm (1 in) and 5 cm (2 in)
- Adhesive plaster (Elastoplast etc) 2.5 and 5 cm
- Cotton wool
- Cotton wool buds
- Sterile dressings, including cotton gauze pads of various sizes
- A thermometer and suitable lubricant
- Feline-safe disinfectant (preferably obtained after advice from your vet)
- Oral dosing syringes, 5 ml and 2 ml
- Pen torch and hand magnifying glass are useful additions.
- Ensure that either on, or in,

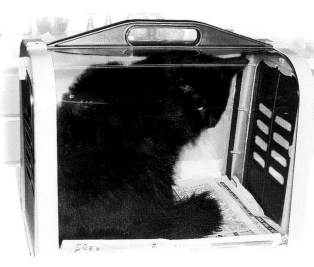

A secure travelling container is essential when you need to get your cat to the vet.

the box are contact details of your vet and transport facilities.

FIRST-AID PROCEDURES

ABSCESSES AND BITE WOUNDS

Cats never need to go outside to develop an abscess. For example, facial abscesses can occur due to scratching as a result of ear irritation.

The first sign is often that the cat is quiet and has a swelling at the site of infection. Bite wounds are usually the result of fighting; they occur commonly on the face or around the tail and rear end (if the cat has been running away!). If left, these often appear to heal but frequently will develop into an abscess in a few days.

If the abscess has not ruptured, take your cat to the vet

without delay. If there is a wound (or the abscess has burst), try to clean the area by gently clipping the hair from around the site. Then bathe with a safe disinfectant. Leave the wound open and consult your vet as soon as possible.

BANDAGING

Cuts and wounds can occur in the home as a result of broken glass and crockery, and outside due to injuries caused by fences, thorns, fights and road accidents.

Try to clean the wound, clipping the hair as necessary with the blunt-ended scissors. If bleeding profusely, bandage the wound if possible.

Bandaging and cats do not go well together!

Most first-aid bandages are applied to control bleeding, usually due to cuts on limbs or torn claws. 5 cm (2 in) bandages are probably the most useful. If conscious, most cats are usually impossible to bandage single-handed. Get help and, if necessary, wrap the cat in a towel, blanket or even a coat. Make sure you secure the bandage in place with adhesive plaster, which should be attached to the hair above the bandage. Always obtain veterinary advice. Even small wounds are often infected and can result in a nasty abscess.

BURNS AND SCALDS

Kittens, and some adult cats, are inquisitive and great chewers. Some seem obsessed with electrical cables, which can be dangerous. In practice, I have seen some horrific burn injuries to the mouth as a result of chewing live electric cables. Flexible cable covers are readily available from most computer stores. These work well as a preventative measure.

If your cat has received a mouth injury, first-aid treatment will be resolutely resisted. Take the cat to the vet ASAP.

If the burn is due to caustic chemicals, try to rinse with plenty of clean, cool water. If the coat is contaminated, clean as much as possible with ordinary soap and water and attempt to prevent licking by wrapping the cat in a towel or blanket. Seek professional help.

EYE INJURIES

These are not uncommon with cats. Bushes, brambles and other cats can be responsible outdoors, as well as injuries due to grass awns and other foreign bodies. Indoors, eye injuries can also happen – particularly in multi-cat households, or when a kitten is introduced to an adult cat. Clipping the front claws of the cats will reduce the risk. *Your vet will show you how.*

Try to bathe the eye with cold water or contact lens solution. If

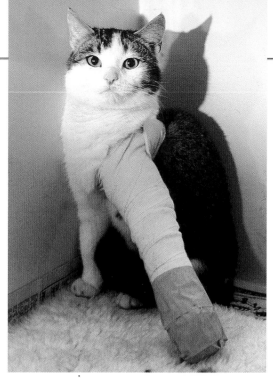

A cat that has been bandaged and splinted following an injury to the foreleg. (Cats and bandages do not go well together!)

there is a penetrating wound, *take the cat to the vet immediately*. If a grass awn or seed appears to be 'floating' on the surface, try to wash it off with drops of water or contact lens solution. If this is successful and the eye appears normal, it is still advisable to seek a vet's opinion. Sometimes the end of the awn can be grasped with tweezers and lifted from the eye.

FITS

These do occur in cats and are always very frightening for the observer. Injuries to the head, plus liver and kidney disease are among possible causes.

Try not to move the cat while in the fit. Try to reduce the amount of light, and turn off any sources of noise, e.g. radio, TV, washing machine etc. Once the

convulsion is over, it is advisable to confine the cat in a suitable box or carrier and take it to your vet as soon as possible for a check in order to establish the cause.

FOREIGN BODIES

This is a veterinary term for anything from a grass awn in the eye or ear to a needle in the stomach.

Grass awns in the eye often lodge under the third eyelid (nictitating membrane). Sometimes it is possible to take hold of the protruding end and lift it away from under the third eyelid. If the eye is tightly closed and any handling of the head is violently resented, *take the cat to the vet without delay.*

It is relatively uncommon for grass seeds to enter the ear of the cat. Ticks, however, sometimes attach to the ears and cause distress. They appear like small, grey warts. Do not be tempted to pull them off. If you do, you are likely to leave the mouth-parts embedded at the site and a slow-healing abscess could result. Surgical spirit or flea spray on some cotton wool held over the tick usually results in the release of the mouth-parts so that it can be removed without a problem.

Foreign bodies in the bowel are not uncommon; often pieces of plastic from children's toys are swallowed. Although some plastics are safe for children, they are often toxic for cats. Vomiting

PART I

and diarrhoea together with lack of appetite are the usual signs.

It is a fact that needles are frequently swallowed by cats. Those without any thread are probably more dangerous since the danger of penetrating the bowel and vital organs is much greater. If thread is present, it will pull the needle through the bowel, and tends to limit the damage. *These are problems that need rapid veterinary help.*

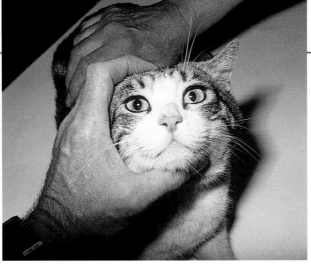

Careful examination is required when injuries occur.

FUR BALLS

Cats are great groomers, and even shorthaired cats swallow large quantities of their loose hair. The feline alimentary tract is designed to cope, usually by vomiting, but sometimes this will not resolve the problem. Partial or complete obstruction due to hair (fur) balls is a well-known clinical entity.

Signs are the same as with other bowel obstructions – lassitude, lack of appetite and vomiting. If the cat is unwell, contact your vet without delay. Early treatment often avoids surgery if hair balls are the cause.

HEAT STROKE

Heat stroke, also known as heat exhaustion or hyperthermia, does occur with cats. It is not as common as with dogs, although the heat control mechanism is similar. Sometimes hyperthermia will occur if the cat is confined in a modern plastic cat carrier in hot weather, especially if stressed, as when being taken to the vet.

The first signs are persistent mouth breathing – panting. Acting on these first signs will often avoid serious consequences. Remember, mouth breathing (panting) does not occur with cats as frequently as with dogs.

Wrap the cat in wet towels or spray with cold water. Increase ventilation as much as you can. If you are in a car, place the carrier near to an open window so there is as much air circulation as possible.

POISONS

Excess salivation, vomiting, diarrhoea and nervous signs, including convulsions and coma, are all signs of poisoning.

If there is contamination of the coat, try to remove as much as possible with plain soap and water or even plain water. Do not use chemical solvents. Tar and creosote in the coat can be removed with warm cooking oil rubbed in, and then mopped off with tissues.

If you think the cat has eaten something poisonous, contact your vet as soon as possible. Vomiting can be induced with salt or mustard on the back of the tongue, but it should not be done until veterinary advice has been received. Remember that many readily available human drugs, such as aspirin and paracetamol, can be toxic to cats.

CLAW DAMAGE

If you have an elderly cat, do be aware that, due to stiffness, claws cannot be retracted as easily as when young. In consequence, their claws can get caught in soft furnishings and result in painful torn claws as the cat tries to get free. Occasional trimming of the tips of the nails is good prevention. Your vet will show you how.

WASHING MACHINES AND DRIERS

Cats are inquisitive and the interiors of washing machines and driers are irresistible. Clothes in the machine make a comfortable bed for any cat seeking solitude. Unfortunately, when the machine is functioning, the results can be horrific. Vigilance is the name of the game.

Always make sure that the interior of these machines is checked before and after use and the door is kept closed.

TIPS FOR GIVING MEDICINE

Chapter 5

PART I

Medicating even the most placid cat can sometimes be an almost impossible task! Therefore, get your cat used to unusual handling from the beginning. Check mouth, ears, eyes and the back end – the same applies whether you have acquired a tiny kitten or an adult cat – although the task will be much easier if you are starting off with a kitten. Practice makes perfect and, believe it or not, cats are creatures of habit so the familiar is not resented.

ROLE PLAY

In order to get your cat used to these intrusive procedures, make them part of the daily 'attention routine' when playing, grooming, or feeding. With the cat or kitten on your knees, place a hand over the head. Then lightly grip the upper jaw and, with the other hand, place either a finger or your thumb on the lower jaw and press gently downwards. The cat will instinctively open its mouth and usually, as quickly, shut it, but that is mission achieved – it will have given you time to have a look. You can do the same thing with the ears as part of the playing or grooming routine: just gently take hold of the pinna (ear flap) and hold it, then have a look down the ear canal, which, incidentally, should be clean with little evidence of wax.

Cats are usually quite sensitive about their private parts and resent interference in that area. Observe the same procedure. As part of the attention routine, grip the base of the tail quite firmly and just take a quick look at the nether regions. Repeat it a few times. You will find that the cat will accept all these strange procedures as part of a game, particularly if young and playful.

Always reward with praise, a favourite game or a delicious food treat!

The next stage is to take a pill-sized treat, ensuring it is food your cat really craves, and repeat the procedure. Open the mouth and this time push the morsel down the throat. Great care is necessary here, particularly if you are doing it for the first time with an adult cat. Cats normally carry bacteria in the mouths, including Pasteurella, which can cause very serious infections in humans. Therefore it is important to avoid being bitten at all costs.

If you foresee problems, ensure you carry out the procedure with competent help. Wrap the cat in a towel or blanket with the head exposed. Your assistant should hold the cat over the shoulders and gently press down so that the front legs cannot be brought up in defence. This will allow you to open the mouth, and drop the

27

PART I

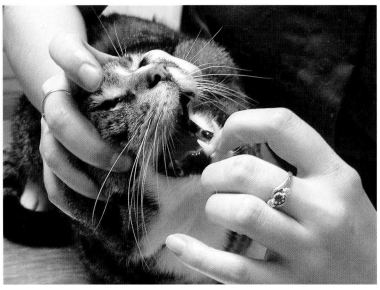

If you practise with treats, it will make it easier when you need to give a tablet.

pill or food morsel at the back of the throat. Then, if necessary, gently push with the back of a smooth pencil or ball pen. Quickly shut the mouth and rub the throat to ensure that the 'pill' is swallowed.

Practising with food morsels makes essential medication a very much easier task when the time comes. It is important throughout to maintain a confident, unstressed approach. Cats can sense our emotions probably better than we can, and will react adversely if they think you are getting upset.

MEDICATION WITHOUT REHEARSAL

If you have not had the opportunity to simulate medication before the actual act is forced on you, so to speak, it is

wise to make a few preparations.
• Get competent, even if not experienced, help.
• Make sure you have a suitable towel or blanket in which to wrap or even roll your cat.
• Ensure the pill is out of the container and near to hand.
• Have a suitable pencil or ball pen ready to aid the ingestion process!
• Finally, don't forget to give lots of fuss – a favourite treat or praise – when the task is successfully accomplished.

GIVING MEDICINE

If you have difficulty with tablets, the vet will very often exchange the medication for a liquid. Feline medication manufacturers are working very hard to produce feline palatable, small-volume, liquid medications, which do

make the job at least a bit easier.

Many of these medicines are also dispensed with specially graduated syringes, which help with accuracy and ease of administration. Even if a syringe is not supplied, your veterinary surgeon will provide one if requested. They are also available from pet outlets.

Often owners find that liquid medicines are easier to administer than pills since, when using a syringe, the mouth need not be opened. The end of the syringe is inserted at the side of the mouth, between the teeth. However, it is important to have competent help holding the cat over the shoulders, allowing you to hold the head from above and raise it into a vertical position. In that way, the lower jaw sags so that the syringe can be inserted without force.

If you have no luck with this procedure, try 'scruffing' the cat – but only as a last resort. One person takes a firm grasp of the loose skin at the back of the neck while the front legs and body are wrapped in the towel or blanket. Place the cat on a table or work top, and press gently downwards, allowing the other person to hold the head vertically and then proceed as before.

Once the medicine has been placed at the back of the throat, rub the marker pads just in front of the ears and, at the same time, keep the mouth closed. If necessary, gently press the nostrils momentarily. This usually results in the cat

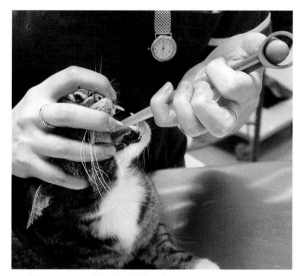

A pill popper makes the job a lot easier.

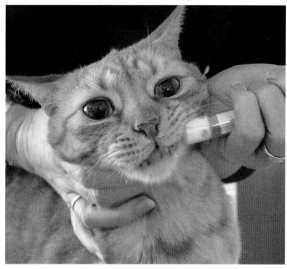

Using a syringe to give fluids.

swallowing very quickly.

You will have noticed that I have omitted the obvious – putting the medication in the food. In my experience, this seldom works. Cats are inordinately suspicious and if they think their food has, in any way, been adulterated, they are prepared to starve. By all means give it a try, but do take note of the fact that most tablets intended for cats are usually coated to improve flavour, and if they are crushed they may be even more unpalatable. Sadly, my experience is that if medicine is unpalatable, diluting it with delicious food just ruins the food as far as the cat is concerned.

CATS FROM HELL
Some cats, despite all the preparation, training and your best efforts still fight tooth and claw if pilling is proposed. Today, vets and many pet shops stock 'pill poppers'. These are plastic gadgets that help with getting the tablet safely down the cat's throat. The pill can be placed in the gadget, the cat's mouth opened and by depressing the plunger, the pill goes down the throat. I can thoroughly recommend them. They are great stress relievers!

It is worth remembering that, as part of feline health care programmes, most cats need worm tablets at least twice a year, so a pill popper is a sound investment.

Do not be afraid to discuss any problems with your vet. It is my experience that the majority of cats can be tableted once or twice a day. If more frequently, it very often it becomes a nightmare procedure. Do not think this is any failure on your part. Discuss it with your vet to see if an alternative medication routine can be worked out.

ADMINISTRATION OF DROPS OR OINTMENTS

EYE DROPS
These are probably easier to apply than ointment. The technique is similar to giving medication. Have someone hold the cat, gently exerting pressure over the shoulders. Take the head from above and with a dropper a few centimetres (an inch or two) above the eye, release one drop into the eye. If the eye is tightly closed, use your forefinger and thumb to gently spread the lids at the same as you place the drops.

Unless instructed to the contrary by your vet, it is always worthwhile applying a drop to the sound eye in the

PART I

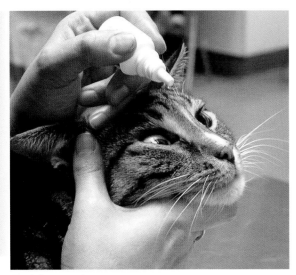

Applying eye drops.

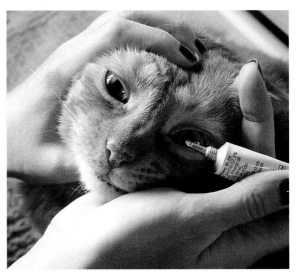

Applying eye ointment.

first place. This will get the cat used to the procedure and it will be less likely to be upset.

EYE OINTMENT

The application of ointment to the eye involves keeping the tube parallel to the eye. With the nozzle pointing to the inner corner, squeeze the ointment along the line of the lids. It does not matter if the eye is closed at this stage because, once the ointment is on the lids, gently stroking your finger across the closed lids will encourage opening and ensure some ointment enters the eye.

EAR DROPS

Many cats need ear preparations, usually applied in the form of drops. These are frequently to remove excess wax, or more usually to eradicate ear mites (*Otodectes cyanotes*). Follow your vet's instructions regarding application. Ear drops are usually supplied either with a separate dropper, or in a plastic bottle – the nozzle of which acts as a dropper. All that is necessary is to squeeze the bottle once the lid has been removed.

Introduce either the nozzle or the tip of the dropper into the top of the external ear canal, and squeeze in a small amount. Gently massage just below the ear to make sure the drops are dispersed. Most cats are quite amenable to this procedure but, as with all feline medication, another pair of hands is a great asset.

FLEA SPRAYS

Most cats instinctively dislike flea sprays, no matter whether they are self-pressurised or of the pump variety. If you have help, it is often easier to put the cat on a table or work top, placing a towel over the head. This restricts sound and sight to some extent, and also protects the head from the spray. Follow the manufacturer's instructions on the pack regarding application.

If your cat is seriously upset by this procedure, discuss with your vet the possibility of using other types of flea control, e.g. spot-on preparations. These only involve the application of a few drops of a special liquid at the back of the neck after the hair has been parted. Some preparations are also available for routine worming.

PART II

COMMON DISEASE PROBLEMS

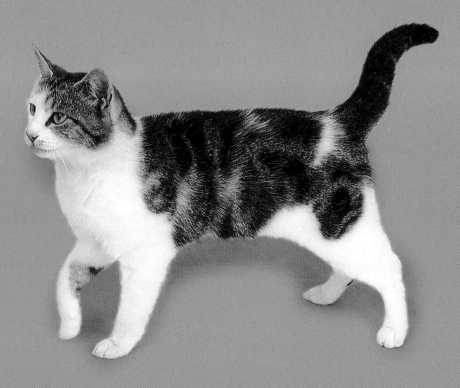

THE EYE (SIGHT)

Chapter 6

There are a number of conditions that affect various parts of the eye. In some cases, these may affect the cat's ability to see.

THE EYELIDS

One of the main functions of the eyelid is to protect the eyeball. Many conditions affecting the eyeballs can be reflected in the appearance of the eyelids, and it is important always to ascertain if the eyeball is affected. This can sometimes be difficult if the eyelids are tightly closed. Wrapping the cat in a towel or blanket, with another pair of hands to aid with restraint, is usually effective to allow gentle parting of the lids to find out if the condition is confined solely to the lids or affects the eyeball itself. If the eyeball condition is very painful, every approach will be resented without

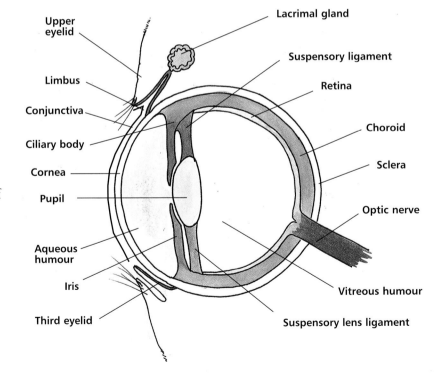

Upper eyelid
Lacrimal gland
Suspensory ligament
Limbus
Retina
Conjunctiva
Ciliary body
Choroid
Cornea
Sclera
Pupil
Optic nerve
Aqueous humour
Iris
Vitreous humour
Third eyelid
Suspensory lens ligament

STRUCTURE OF THE EYE

sedation/analgesia. Even if the white of the eye only appears red and sore, it is probably better at this stage to seek help from your vet.

BLEPHARITIS

Swelling (inflammation) in the eyelids is known as blepharitis. This is not uncommon in younger cats. It usually also affects other parts of the eye.
Treatment: If it just appears that the lids are suddenly sore, provided the cat is not rubbing them too much and making the condition worse, try bathing with cold water or saline (contact lens solution). If there is not an improvement in an hour or so, you should contact your vet, since, if the problem continues, self-inflicted damage to the eyeball is very likely.

CYSTS AND OTHER GROWTHS

Cysts and other small growths on the eyelids also occur. These tend to be seen more commonly in the older cat and often require surgery.

GRASS AWNS AND OTHER FOREIGN BODIES

In summertime particularly, it is not uncommon for a cat that spends part of the day outside to come home with a tightly closed eye. Usually any attempts to open the eyelids are strongly resented, and the likelihood is that there is a grass awn, thorn, or other foreign body lying

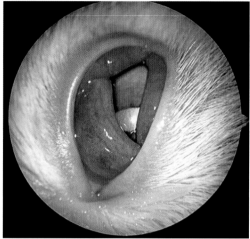

Conjunctivitis.

beneath the lids. This can potentially cause injury and great pain to the eyeball itself.
Treatment: An urgent trip to the vet will be necessary so that the cat can be sedated, or even anaesthetised, in order to examine the eye and treat appropriately.

Inflammation resulting not only in blepharitis, but also affecting the eyeball, i.e conjunctivitis (inflammation of the thin, transparent membrane covering the eyeball, see next section), can be due to viruses and secondary bacterial infection, particularly those involved with cat flu. Some of these can be very serious, and therefore prompt veterinary assistance is a priority, especially in the young kitten.
Inflammation confined solely to the eyelids, on the other hand, can often be due to an allergic response, such as a reaction to pollen, some other plant allergy, or an insect sting. In 'indoor

cats' this type of reaction can be due to cleaning agents, such as washing powder, carpet cleaners etc.

THE EYEBALL

There are many relatively common conditions affecting the cat's eye.

CONJUNCTIVITIS

This is inflammation of the very thin, normally transparent membrane, which lines the eyelid and also covers the eye itself. The most common cause is infection, but it can also be due to an allergy, e.g. some cats are sensitive to certain pollens, hair sprays etc. Irritation from a foreign body, e.g. a grass awn or piece of dirt beneath the lids, will also cause this reaction. Another common cause is contact with irritant substances, such as flea spray or shampoo, that has accidentally got into the eye.
Signs: The immediate reaction is an increase in tears and blood flow to the tissue so the cat appears to have a watery, red eye. If infected or neglected, this soon turns to a pussy discharge. In kittens particularly, this often dries and gums the eyelids together so that the poor kitten is incapable of opening them.
Treatment: Gentle bathing with a little warm water will often 'ungum' the lids, allowing examination of the eyeball. If the condition continues, veterinary treatment will be required, probably involving antibiotics and special eye drops.

PART II

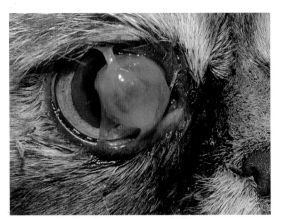

Corneal rupture following a cat fight.

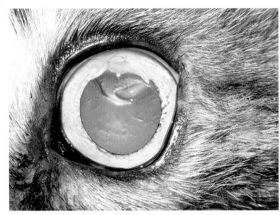

Corneal ulceration following a cat fight.

CORNEAL WOUNDS AND ULCERS

The cornea is the clear area in the front of the eye through which light passes, allowing sight. Injury to this area is not uncommon. Cats that normally spend time outside can injure the cornea as a result of scratches from bushes in the garden, or from other cats. Grass awns and other foreign bodies lodged under the eyelids can result in extremely painful corneal ulcers in a very short time.

Signs: The cat presents with a tightly closed eye and will resent any handling of the face. If left untreated, the ulcer can deepen and the eyeball may rupture and collapse, which can result in loss of the eye.

Treatment: Veterinary attention is urgent. Under sedation or general anaesthesia the eye will be examined. Sometimes surgery is required.

GLAUCOMA

Ageing cats can suffer from glaucoma, just like us. This is the name given to the condition that results from increased pressure within the eyeball.

Signs: If very slow in onset, it does not bother the cat initially and often the first sign is that the affected eye appears larger than the other.

Treatment: Today there are several treatments available that successfully control this condition. If left untreated glaucoma will lead to blindness, the affected eye often having to be removed to relieve pain due to the ever-increasing pressure.

CATARACTS

Suspended within the eye is a crystalline transparent lens that concentrates the light rays on the retina (the light-sensitive surface at the back of the eye). Sometimes this lens becomes cloudy, which interferes with vision.

One of the most common causes of cataract in the cat is damage to the lens. This can be due to trauma, penetrating wounds or inflammation within the eye. Often cataract results due to dislocation of the lens within the eye.

Sugar diabetes (Diabetes mellitus) is another cause. This condition is not uncommon in the cat.

Signs: Older cats will sometimes have 'opaque looking' eyes in reflected light. This does not necessarily mean that they have cataracts, or that they are blind. It merely indicates that the lens has contracted with age, giving it a grey, dense appearance. The condition is known as senile sclerosis. Often light can still pass through the lens to the back of the eye so that vision is not impaired too much. However, if you are at all concerned, consult your vet.

Treatment: If the lens has dislocated, you may be referred to a specialist veterinary ophthalmologist. In the cat, cataract surgery involving the removal of the lens is a very specialised operation, but can restore sight to the eye.

THE EAR (HEARING)

Chapter 7

The external appearance of the ear, irrespective of breed, is relatively standard in the cat. Dogs, in contrast, show enormous breed variance – ears can be pricked or dropped, relatively hairless or completely enveloped in hair. The only breed of cat with a non-standard ear is the Scottish Fold. Unlike longhaired dogs, where the amount of hair on the head and on the actual ear flap itself often obscures the ear from sight, longhaired cats (Persians) have ears that are covered with hair that is little different from the shorthaired breeds, although they may have a few quite spectacular longer hairs, known as ear furnishings, growing from just within the tip.

In both cats and dogs, the ears are not only involved with sound but also balance – and this can be of greater significance to the

STUCTURE OF THE EAR

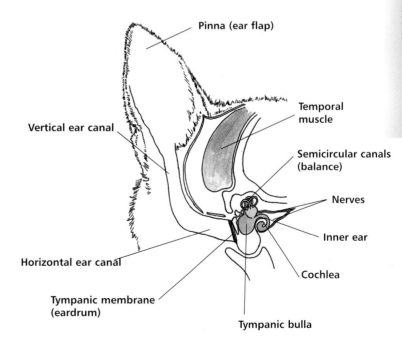

- Pinna (ear flap)
- Temporal muscle
- Semicircular canals (balance)
- Nerves
- Inner ear
- Cochlea
- Tympanic bulla
- Tympanic membrane (eardrum)
- Horizontal ear canal
- Vertical ear canal

cat, who performs far more spectacular balancing acts than even the most daredevil dog!

Despite the fact there is little variation in the appearance of the cat's ears, and they do not suffer from specific disease problems associated with pendulous floppy ears like those of spaniels, nevertheless ear problems are relatively commonplace in cats.

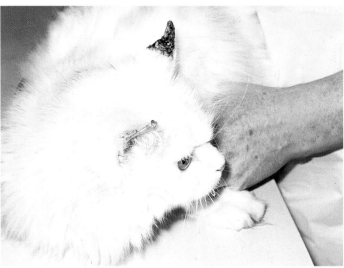

Tumour and necrosis on the left ear tip; right ear affected with solar dermatitis.

ANATOMY OF THE EAR

The ear flap, which projects from the upper part of the head, is only a very small part of the complex organ known as the ear. The pinna, or ear flap, is part of the external ear, which channels sounds down a tunnel in the side of the face. This tube turns inwards towards the ear drum (tympanum). On the other side of this are the middle and inner ears concerned with the passage of sound and also balance. Thus, although part of the external ear can be seen, this is only a small part; the other structures are hidden from view, deep inside the skull.

Nerve endings in the inner ear transmit electrical impulses generated by sound waves to the hearing centre in the brain. Not surprisingly, such a complicated structure can have problems.

OTITIS

Inflammation of any part of the ear is known as otitis; consequently, this is divided into **otitis externa**, **media** and **interna**, depending on which part of the ear is affected. Otitis externa, inflammation of the outer part of the ear, is by far the most common. Causes include ear mites, excess wax, irritation from foreign bodies such as grass awns, as well as infection with bacteria and fungae. Some types of cancer, particularly polyps, may also be implicated.

Signs: Shaking and rubbing; sometimes a discharge and smell.

Treatment: Examination will probably require general anaesthesia to remove wax and other debris. Your vet may prescribe drops that will not only eradicate the mites and any

secondary infection, but also alleviate the soreness and prevent the build-up of further wax.

EAR MITES AND WAX

Part of regular grooming should always include inspection of the external ear canal for signs of any mites or wax. Ear mites are just visible to the naked eye. Vets use an instrument called an auriscope (otoscope), which is essentially a specially shaped, illuminated magnifying glass made to go down the external ear canal. With this instrument, mites and other problems can be diagnosed relatively easily.

Mites are picked up from other cats; kittens will often acquire them from their mother while still in the nest. Mites feed on the ear wax, which, in an attempt to reduce the irritation caused by the tiny mites, is produced in even greater quantities. Thus a vicious circle is soon set up.

Signs: Many cats will carry ear mites without them apparently causing problems, but it should be remembered that they will be passed on to other cats and to dogs, where they can cause considerably more irritation than they do in the average cat.

Excess wax, which is often a

dark brownish-black colour, helps even the most novice owner realise there is something the matter with the ears. The cat tends to rub and scratch so that secondary infection and a chronic external otitis soon occurs. **Treatment:** Simple treatment involving the use of a few drops of medicinal paraffin (liquid paraffin) or 'anti-mite' drops,

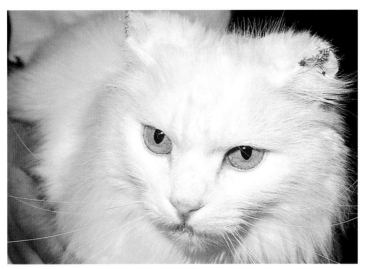

Post-operative, following amputation of the ear flaps.

obtainable from any pet supplies outlet, works well if the condition is noticed early enough. However, if the ear appears very red and sore, or there is a great deal of excess wax, a visit to the vet is advisable.

AURAL HAEMATOMA

Also known as a blood blister, this is quite a common condition in cats, particularly those with ear irritation (e.g. ear mites). The ear flap (pinna) consists of a supporting cartilage covered on both sides by skin. Blood vessels run just beneath the skin and vigorous shaking and rubbing can cause some of these tiny vessels to break and bleed, resulting in a blood blister. This, in turn, worries the cat, which results in more shaking and rubbing. The injured vessel continues to bleed under the skin, and thus the blister, known as a haematoma,

gets bigger. With all but the smallest haematomata, cure depends upon surgical intervention by the vet.

CANCER

Tumours of the pinna arise from the skin and these are not uncommon in white cats. They are often located on the tip of the ear. Most commonly they are due to the development of a squamous cell carcinoma (SCC), which, as in humans, is related to exposure to sunlight and lack of protective pigment in the skin (melanin).

Signs: Usually the first signs are that the ear tip appears scabby, sore and ulcerated and seems thicker than normal. Occasionally there is a proliferative lumpy growth that bleeds easily. If recognised early enough, medical treatment can be effective. This involves the use

of sun blocks and careful control to ensure the cat does not lie out in strong sunlight. **Treatment:** The majority of these ear tumours do eventually need surgery, which may involve total amputation of the ear flap. This sounds horrendous but in most cases is completely curative. Perhaps, on reflection, if the cat just had a little more hair on the ear flap, like its canine friends, such major surgery would not be necessary!

FOREIGN BODIES IN THE EXTERNAL AUDITORY CANAL

The most usual foreign bodies in cats' ears are grass awns, seeds etc. In practice, I also had one or two cases of cats that have had beads and other tiny objects put in their ears by small children. Depending on the cat's temperament, the presence of anything within the ear canal usually results in violent shaking and rubbing, which can eject the object, but usually only makes the situation worse – hence a trip to the vet will be necessary.

Treatment: This will often require a general anaesthetic to examine the ear canal and remove the foreign body.

PART II

INFECTIONS OF THE SKIN OF THE EAR

It should not be forgotten that the ear flap and the lining of the external ear canal are parts of the skin, and thus any skin diseases (see page 43) can affect the ear. Ringworm, which is caused by a fungus, (e.g. Microsporum canis), is the most common problem.

Some allergy-prone cats will also show allergic reactions involving the ears, which will often become bright red in a matter of minutes when in contact with the particular substance causing the allergy (allergen). In cats this is not infrequently some form of pollen.

MIDDLE EAR PROBLEMS

OTITIS MEDIA

This is an infection of the middle ear, which usually arises as the result of infection of the external ear canal (otitis externa) that has passed through the ear drum (tympanic membrane). However, there is a tube (Eustachian tube) which extends between the throat and the middle ear. Its function is to equalise the pressure on the two sides of the delicate ear drum. Sometimes cats with chronic throat infections can end

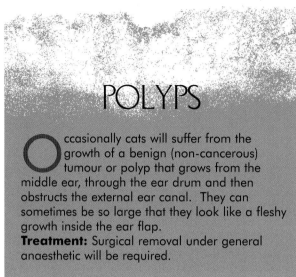

POLYPS

Occasionally cats will suffer from the growth of a benign (non-cancerous) tumour or polyp that grows from the middle ear, through the ear drum and then obstructs the external ear canal. They can sometimes be so large that they look like a fleshy growth inside the ear flap.
Treatment: Surgical removal under general anaesthetic will be required.

up with middle ear disease due to infection travelling along the Eustachian tube.
Signs: These are similar to external otitis – shaking of the head, scratching at one or both ears, and the cat may show a disinclination to have its head touched. Sometimes there is a head tilt.

INNER EAR PROBLEMS

INHERITED DEAFNESS

Some, but not all, white cats can suffer from an inherited form of deafness particularly if they have blue eyes. This is incurable. It is due to degeneration of structures within the inner ear and is present virtually from birth. Such cats learn to live a normal life, but are at special risk if allowed out, due to traffic, dogs and other animals.

OTITIS INTERNA

Inflammation and infection of the inner ear often occurs as an extension of middle ear disease.
Signs: Usually there is loss of balance rather than loss of hearing. Other signs can include shaking of the head and uncontrollable, rapid eye movement known as nystagmus. In severe cases, cats can fall over when attempting to walk.
Treatment: Treatment for otitis interna can be difficult. Like otitis media, long courses of powerful antibiotics are usually prescribed. Corticosteroids are sometimes also included in an attempt to reduce inflammation. Balance problems are usually slow to recover, but cats seem able to compensate with time.

IDIOPATHIC VESTIBULAR SYNDROME

This a condition of unknown cause that can affect the balance of otherwise perfectly normal cats. There is usually a severe head tilt, incoordination and nystagmus, and no obvious signs of external or middle ear infection. Antibiotics are often prescribed as an insurance against inner ear infection, but many cats recover spontaneously after one to two weeks.

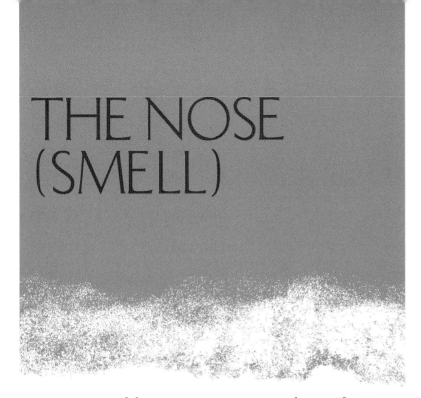

THE NOSE (SMELL)

Chapter 8

Because of the prevalence of flu viruses in cats, nasal problems are not uncommon. In this regard a good take-home message is to ensure that flu vaccinations are completed as early as possible, and regular boosters are always administered according to veterinary recommendation (see Chapter Two).

There are several signs that indicate a possible nasal problem, although individually they are not specific for any particular disease. Overall, however, they may give an indication of the problem.

The signs are nasal discharge, sneezing and, if the nasal cavities are blocked, open-mouth breathing. Unlike dogs, cats do not normally 'pant' as a mechanism for heat loss, except in exceptional circumstances, e.g. extreme heat or if very stressed. If your cat appears to be frequently mouth breathing for no apparent reason, discuss it with your vet.

PROBLEMS ON THE OUTSIDE OF THE NOSE

Anything affecting the outside of the nose is unlikely to affect the sense of smell. There are two conditions that affect the rhinarium, which is the hairless skin surrounding the nostrils of the cat.

CANCER

The most common form is **squamous cell carcinoma (SCC).** This, as with the ear, most commonly affects white-nosed cats. It starts just as a small ulcer, which will quickly grow to involve both nostrils. Then, of course, the sense of smell can be seriously affected.

Squamous cell tumours in this site are much more difficult to remove than those on the ear (see page 37) so, if in doubt, consult your vet without delay.

ULCERATION

Extensive ulceration can affect the outside of the nose. This is often not cancerous, but is due to an auto-immune problem as a result of which the cat produces antibodies against its own nasal tissues. Treatment usually involves the use of corticosteroids for this unpleasant condition.

TRAUMA

The outside of nose can also be injured in accidents, particularly in fights with other cats. These usually take the form of superficial scratches, but sometimes can be more severe. **Treatment:** Usually antibiotics and analgesics (painkillers) are prescribed.

PROBLEMS INSIDE THE NOSE

Infection of the nasal cavity can be due to viral, bacterial or fungal causes. All result in inflammation, which, in the nose, is called **rhinitis**.

RHINITIS

Feline herpes virus (FHV) and feline calicivirus (FCV) are the two main agents involved in so-called 'cat flu' and are frequently the cause of infected rhinitis. Secondary bacterial infection can often lead to chronic rhinitis, the medical term for 'snotty nose' syndrome. Despite the wide use of flu vaccines, cat flu is still common and the viruses are very widespread (see Chapter Two).

Although specific antiviral agents are becoming available for use in cats, treatment, particularly in the early stages of the disease, still mainly depends on good nursing care. This often has to be carried out by the owner. Antibiotics are frequently required on an intermittent basis to prevent secondary bacterial infection.

Unfortunately, even with the best nursing, some cats become chronic 'snufflers'. These cats often have seriously impaired taste and smell. Chronic 'snufflers' often have recurrent, acute attacks. During these attacks, the cat actually sheds virus and is infectious to any other susceptible cats with which it is in contact.

When having an acute attack, the cat is frequently off its food because it can neither smell nor taste it. Therefore, the provision of strong-smelling and tasting foods often gets the cat over the attack more quickly by getting it eating once more. The choice of food obviously depends on the cat, but strong-smelling fish, prawns etc. are the usual favourites.

Bear in mind that vaccination does not prevent infection, but does reduce the signs (symptoms) of the disease.

Bacteria are often involved as secondary invaders, particularly when there is a viral rhinitis. However, one bacteria, *Chlamydophyla psittaci* (previously known as *Chamydia psittaci*) can cause disease on its own. A vaccine is available which is useful in situations of risk (see Chapter Two).

Fungal infections can also occur but are probably more common in North America than

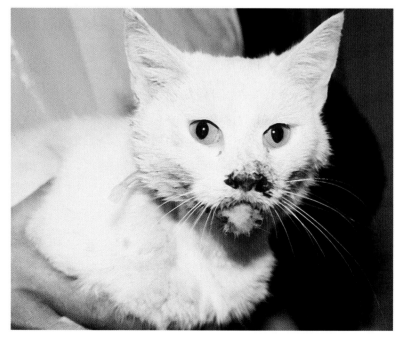

Nasal injuries following a road traffic accident. (The cat has a pharyngostomy tube in place for feeding until the injury heals.)

PART II

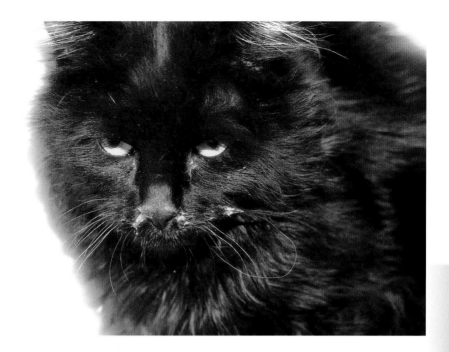

Chronic rhinitis – note the discharge from the nostrils.

in the UK. *Cryptococcus neoformans* is the fungal organism most commonly involved. Skin, eyes and nervous tissue can also be affected. It is often associated with infections involving FIV and FeLV.

Foreign bodies, particularly blades of grass, often find their way into the noses of cats. The usual signs are sudden violent sneezing attacks. The problem is that not all the grass is removed as a result of sneezing. This can lead to chronic rhinitis and permanent impairment of the sense of smell. If in doubt, consult your vet as early as possible.

POLYPS

Polyps have already been mentioned in respect of growing into the ear. (see page 38). Sometimes, although arising from the same site, the polyp grows in the other direction and ends up in the back of the throat. Difficult breathing, sneezing and a nasal discharge are the result. Surgical removal is the only remedy that is likely to be permanent.

THE TONGUE (TASTE)

Chapter 9

Problems do occur with the feline tongue, but, compared with other sense organs, these are few. They include the following:

CORROSIVE OR BURN INJURIES

Although fastidious in their habits, cats occasionally make mistakes and lick corrosive and irritant substances, e.g. bleach, battery acid, etc. As a result they can damage the tongue, causing glossitis (inflammation), and occasionally permanent taste problems can result.

Signs: Profuse salivation and difficulty in swallowing are the main signs.

Treatment: Veterinary treatment is required because often the cat is unable to drink until healing has taken place. Depending on the severity of the injury, antibiotics and analgesics will be required, and often,

subsequently, corticosteroids to reduce the amount of scarring.

TRAUMA

Injuries to the tongue are not uncommon, particularly in feral and semi-feral cats as a result of licking open food cans. Occasionally injuries can be acquired while fighting.

Signs: These are similar to corrosive or burn injuries, with the addition that there may often be copious haemorrhage.

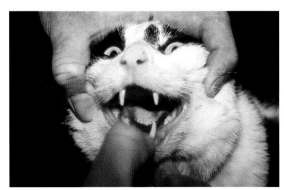

Caustic burns on the tongue.

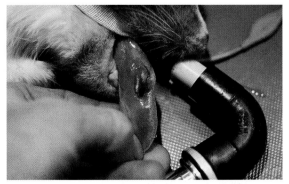

This cat has a tumour of the tongue, which is quite rare.

THE SKIN (TOUCH)

10 Chapter

F ew of us tend to think of the skin as a body organ like the liver, heart or kidneys. It is, in fact, the largest organ of the body and has a number of functions essential to life, just as important as any of the other essential organs.

- The skin forms a barrier between the cat and its environment and acts against physical and chemical damage.
- It inhibits infection with micro-organisms – bacteria, fungi and viruses. (see Chapter Nineteen).
- It has an important function in conserving water and minerals essential for the body.
- It is involved in the regulation of body temperature.

Among all its other functions, the skin can be regarded as an organ of special sense since it

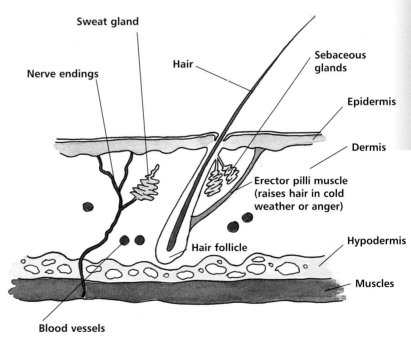

STRUCTURE OF THE SKIN

43

houses the sensory nerves responsible for touch. Damage to these nerves can result in areas becoming devoid of sensation. If this affects the foot pads, for example, cuts, burns and scalds can then result without the cat being aware.

In addition to the paw pads, receptors in the tip of the nose are known to be able to determine the difference between warmth and cold. The cat's whiskers, properly known as the vibrissae, grow out stiffly from the side of the muzzle and are important sensory organs. In addition to these specialised hairs, guard hairs all over the cat's skin contain touch receptors, which will indicate the nearness of objects that the cat cannot see.

Skin disease in cats is relatively common, usually due to fleas and other ectoparasites.

PROBLEMS WITH FLEAS
(see page 18)
If there is very heavy flea infestation, it is thought that the movement of the adult fleas on the cat in search of food can be a source of irritation to the cat. Most of the problems, however, are the result of an allergic reaction to flea saliva injected when the flea feeds on the cat. This leads to intense itching, (pruritis), resulting in licking, chewing and scratching by the cat. This self-induced injury will usually become secondarily infected, and an obvious flea allergy dermatitis develops, often

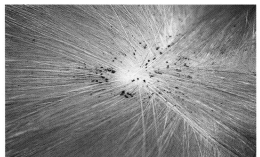

Flea dirt seen on a cat's coat.

with large infected sores and plaques. It is interesting that some non-allergic cats can carry a huge flea burden without any apparent problems.

SIGNS IN ALLERGIC CATS
Depending how allergic the cat is, the lesions can vary from minimal hair loss to a widespread rash with raised, angry-looking sores affecting mainly the base of the tail, the back, the abdomen between the hind legs, and sometimes the face and ears.

DIAGNOSIS
Diagnosis depends on identifying fleas or flea dirt on the coat. In highly sensitive cats, an allergic response can be triggered by the bite of just one flea, which, by the time lesions have occurred, may have left the cat.

Diagnosis can be difficult if, despite careful examination, no fleas are found. This is why cats with skin lesions that may be due to so-called **flea allergy dermatitis (FAD)** are invariably placed on a strict flea control programme initially, even if no

fleas are found. This is always a cause of frustration, if not irritation, to owners if the situation has not been carefully explained or understood when they initially consult their vet.

TREATMENT
Treatment not only involves de-fleaing the cat but – just as importantly – the environment with 'cat-safe' products. This will seem a costly and pointless exercise if the owner has not seen evidence of fleas and does not understand why it is so essential.

PROBLEMS WITH LICE
(See page 19).
Health problems with lice usually only arise in poorly reared, feral or immuno-suppressed cats (e.g. FIV or FeLV positive). However, it should be remembered that kittens are immuno-incompetent, particularly while suckling, and if poorly reared in unhygienic conditions, health problems due to lice infestation can occur.

SIGNS
Since lice are approximately the size of fleas (about 2.5 mm) and move very slowly if at all, they can be easily identified on an infested cat. Intense irritation (pruritis) invariably occurs. In kittens, heavy infestations can cause serious anaemia and even death. In cats, the most usual louse found is *Felicola substratus* (a biting louse).

Lice, like fleas, infest a whole range of animals, including us,

PART II

but they are fairly host-specific. We are unlikely to be bitten by cat lice.

TREATMENT
Control is far easier with lice than fleas since they do not live in the environment. Cat-safe, spot-on or spray preparations are effective, but the manufacturer's instructions on the pack should be carefully followed.

PROBLEMS WITH TICKS
(see page 19)
Ticks are probably more of a problem to cats in North America than in the UK. They carry many diseases, some of which can be communicated to us. They infest the cat in order to obtain a blood meal. In the UK, ticks have recently assumed much greater importance with the introduction of PETS, the Pet Travel Scheme. This allows cats (and dogs) to enter and re-enter the UK from approved countries without undergoing quarantine, provided they fulfil the strict regulations. Many 'foreign' ticks can carry diseases that not only affect our pets but can also cause human disease. These ticks could enter Britain in the hair coat of their feline host. In consequence, cats (and dogs) entering or re-entering Britain under PETS have to receive approved anti-tick treatment between 24-48 hours before entry.

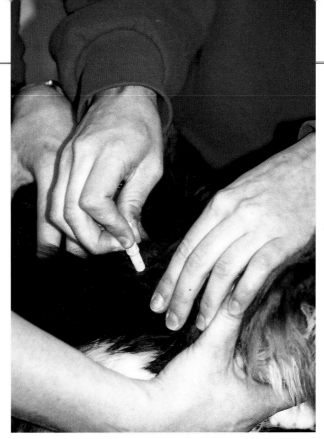
A spot-on treatment can be used to prevent flea infestation.

The main tick-related problem in the UK occurs if the tick is scratched or rubbed off by the cat when attached, or when well-meaning owners try to pull them off. This often results in the mouth-parts being left behind, resulting in a slow-healing wound that can often become infected.

To remove a tick, do not use a lighted cigarette or try to pull it off. Apply flea spray, surgical spirit, or even nail varnish remover to a piece of cotton wool and hold it over the tick for a short period. It can then be safely removed with a twisting motion.

If in doubt, consult your veterinary surgeon, who sell you a tick hook for this purpose.

PROBLEMS WITH MITES
(See page 19)

EAR MITES
Ear mites (*Otodectes cyanotis*) are a common cause of acute ear irritation in the cat (see page 19). Just visible to the naked eye, they are, in the majority of cases, diagnosed by the veterinarian using an auriscope (gloscope). This is an instrument that illuminates and magnifies the ear canal. They can also be diagnosed by laboratory examination of the typically crusty brown/black waxy ear discharge in which they live.
Treatment: Once the cause is confirmed, treatment with anti-parasitic ear drops is usually effective. These can be bought over the counter from the pet store, but ideally should be obtained from your vet, who will be in a better position to prescribe appropriate drops. Often, there is secondary bacterial infection, which will also need treatment. Treatment for the mites must involve all the cats and dogs in the household. Occasionally, with very heavy infestation, mites will also migrate to the hair around the ears, and sometimes to the base of the tail. They infest these areas because a cat will normally curl

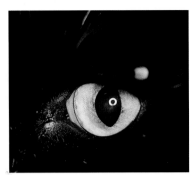

A tick situated above the eye.

up with the head round towards its tail. In these cases, control depends upon the use of anti-parasitic ear drops and an appropriate anti-parasite skin preparation.

"FUR" MITE – CHEYLETIELLOSIS

Cheyletiella ("walking dandruff") mites are not host-specific and are often contracted by cats from rabbits and dogs.

Signs: Walking dandruff is an appropriate name since the *Cheyletiella* mite looks like a tiny bit of dandruff moving between the hairs. *Cheyletiella* mites can sometimes cause much distress to the cat due to pruritis (irritation). This varies with the individual cat.

Treatment: Effective treatment depends on identification of the causal mites by your vet, and the use of a suitable parasiticide, both on the cat and the environment.

NOTOEDRIC MANGE

Feline scabies is fairly rare in cats, but it is very contagious and will spread through litters of kittens very quickly. It is unlikely to cause problems in adult cats, and then only if the cat is immuno-suppressed, e.g. FIV, FeLV positive. Young kittens are immuno-incompetent for the first few weeks of their life, which probably accounts for the rapid spread of notoedric mange if contracted by a litter.

Signs: Early signs in litters are hairlessness and obvious pruritis. In older cats, eczematous lesions may be seen, particularly affecting the ears, head, legs and groin.

Treatment: Treatment of affected cats with any of the feline insecticidal shampoos usually results in rapid improvement. However, diagnosis has to be accurate and usually is the result of laboratory examination of skin scrapings taken by your vet.

HARVEST MITES (Berry bugs)

In certain localities, particularly those with chalky soil both in the UK and the US, this mite infestation can be a problem.

Signs: Signs can vary from a mild dermatitis to severe eczema due to the pruritis. The larval mite is picked up from vegetation. Problems occur mainly in late summer and autumn. Feet, head and ears are usually affected. The larval mites, approximately 0.2 mm can just be seen as bright orange dots on the skin.

Treatment: Treatment with feline-safe anti-parasitic sprays or washes is usually effective.

Wearing a flea collar in the autumn is considered a good preventative measure in areas where the causal mite *Trombicula autunmalis* is prevalent.

RINGWORM

Ringworm is a fungus infection, although often classified as a parasitic condition. It involves non-living parts of the skin, mainly the hair shafts themselves and the dead top layers (stratum corneum) of skin. Occasionally the nails may be involved. This depends on the particular type of ringworm fungus involved.

Ringworm affects many species of animals, including man, and several fungal species can cause problems in cats. The majority of feline cases are due to *Microsporum canis*. Some cats, particularly the longhaired (Persian) breeds, carry the fungus without showing any signs. These asymptomatic carriers are a source of infection to other animals and to us.

SIGNS

Ringworm obtained its name in man because the fungus usually causes circular, very itchy, red areas on the skin. In the cat, diagnosis on physical appearance is not that easy. The skin lesions can vary from an apparent increase in scurf to tiny raised crusty pimples on the skin, so-called **milliary eczema lesions**. These can often be felt more easily than seen. In advanced cases, hairless patches may develop – only very occasionally are these round in shape.

DIAGNOSIS
Positive diagnosis depends on the clinical signs plus the demonstration of *Microsporum canis* by the use of a special ultraviolet lamp (known as Wood's lamp), which causes any infected hairs to fluoresce with an apple green colour. However, this is not totally diagnostic since only about 60 per cent of *Microsporum canis* fluoresce. The "gold standard" is laboratory examination and culture of hair pluckings and brushings. Obviously, if this can be carried out from fluorescing hairs, so much the better.

Ringworm can be a major problem with show cats. If ringworm is suspected at vetting-in at any of the major cat shows held under Governing Council of the Cat Fancy (GCCF) rules in the UK, all cats belonging to the exhibitor have to be rejected from the show. The cats cannot be shown again, and the exhibitor may not attend any future shows, until veterinary examination and tests have shown that the lesions are not caused by ringworm. If the tests are positive, the ban remains in place until two consecutive tests, eight weeks apart, are negative. This can be a very expensive and time-consuming process.

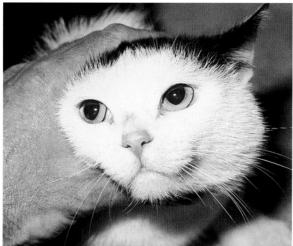

Typical ringworm lesion on the bridge of the nose.

An initial positive diagnosis of ringworm does not have to be made. All that is necessary is for there to be suspicious lesions when the cat is presented at vetting-in. It is prudent always to err on the side of caution. Don't take any cat with any skin problem, however minor, to a show. In Britain, even if such an exhibit is accompanied by a veterinary surgeon's certificate explaining that the problem is not ringworm, the ultimate decision rests with the duty vet and the cat may still be rejected.

TREATMENT
Today we have a variety of antifungal agents that can be used for treatment, but if ringworm is suspected, it is essential that veterinary advice is sought without delay. Treatment always takes weeks rather than days.

ALLERGIC SKIN DISEASE
Cats do suffer form various types of allergic skin disease. These are often the result of hypersensitivity reactions due to an exaggerated response on the part of the cat to the presence of a foreign substance, which in this context is known as an allergen.

Flea saliva has already been mentioned (page 44), but other parasites, foods, drugs, pollens and dust can all result in allergic reactions. The body reacts in an atypical way to the allergen, and this usually results in inflammation. Depending where it occurs, the allergy can take different forms. For example, flea allergies usually result in inflammation of the skin with intense itching and hair loss. Similarly, large wheals – so-called 'nettle rash' – can occur when a cat has brushed against or lain among plants to which it happens to be allergic.

Cats, like people, are not born with allergies. They develop after repeated exposure to the allergen. It is for this reason cats develop food allergy dermatitis, for example, after having been fed that particular diet for many years.

To make diagnosis even more difficult, some cats may be allergic to more than one substance. In addition, they may develop new allergies after previous ones have been controlled. The allergic cat is never an easy case!

PART II

As our knowledge of these sensitivity reactions increases, specific feline allergies have become recognised. Thus, vets now regularly recognise feline dietary allergies. Inhalant allergic reactions in cats were at one time thought to be responsible only for certain types of dermatitis, so-called **atopic dermatitis**. It is now realised that many causes of feline asthma are also due to inhalant allergies see page 69).

Milliary dermatitis or **milliary eczema** is a particularly common 'itchy skin condition' in the cat. The exact cause is still not definitely established, although it does appear to be a hypersensitivity reaction in which fleas and other ectoparasites can play a part, as well as dietary hypersensitivity. Recently, it has been suggested that nutritional deficiencies, such as fatty acids, may also be implicated.

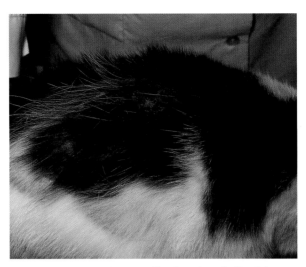

Extensive ringworm lesion, affecting the whole of the right side of the cat.

SIGNS
The cat is generally itchy, and tiny pimples or granules can be felt, if not seen, throughout the cat's fur, particularly along the back and around the neck. These granules, on closer examination, turn out to be little, dried scabs or pimples. As with cases of atopic hypersensitivity, long-term anti-inflammatory drugs are needed to control the problem.

EOSINOPHILIC GRANULOMA COMPLEX
Another complicated feline skin condition is eosinphilic granuloma complex. Granulomas are areas of inflammation, and in the cat can take the form of red, moist, hairless patches on or around the lips. Many different names have been given to the same condition when it occurs in different parts of the body. These include eosinophilic plaque, indolent ulcer, rodent ulcer etc. Today three distinct types of eosinophilic granuloma are recognised.

1. Eosinophilic ulcer, which is used to describe a slow-healing ulcer on the upper lips of the cat.
2. Eosinophilic plaques, which appear as raised, moist, red, ulcerated areas usually on the underside of the abdomen

and inside the thighs.
3. Linear granulomas, which are usually long, thin sore areas. They occur on the backs of the legs, and also sometimes inside the mouth.

The term eosinophilic is used because laboratory examination of many of these plaques and ulcers reveal a high preponderance of a particular type of white blood cell, often associated with allergic conditions and known as an eosinophil.

The cause of eosinophilic granuloma complex is not fully understood. Contributing factors in susceptible cats appear to be flea or food allergies. It does appear that the underlying causes may be the same as those causing milliary dermatitis.

TREATMENT
Treatment involves the use of anti-inflammatory drugs, in particular glucocorticoids, essential fatty acids and antihistamines. These are the mainstays of treatment. Since the cause is not fully understood, treatment in many cases is really only palliative rather than curative; in other words, the condition is just kept under control. Nevertheless, fleas or other parasites should always be vigilantly prevented.

THE MOUTH AND TEETH

11
Chapter

The teeth and mouth of the cat have evolved as a result of the original carnivorous lifestyle. As a result of domestication, particularly associated with the feeding of soft, pre-prepared foods, gum disease, known as periodontal disease, is today a major problem with our cats. A recent survey showed that more than 80 per cent of cats over the age of three years had periodontal disease.

TEETH

It is always worthwhile, wherever possible, getting a kitten used to having its mouth opened so that the teeth can be examined. There are 30 permanent teeth in the cat, 16 in the upper jaw and 14 in the lower jaw. They should all appear white and firmly fixed in the jaw. Any discolouration is usually due to tartar (calculus) and occasionally a damaged or broken tooth.

Tartar (calculus) is not

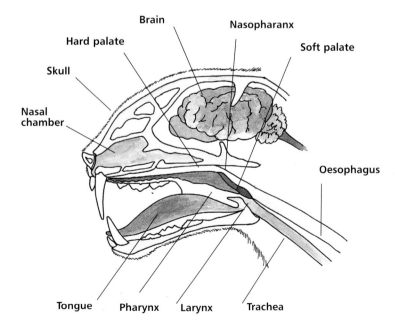

Brain
Nasopharanx
Hard palate
Soft palate
Skull
Nasal chamber
Oesophagus
Tongue
Pharynx
Larynx
Trachea

SECTION THROUGH THE HEAD

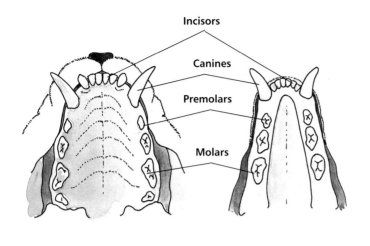

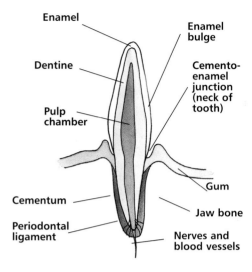

DENTITION

CROSS SECTION OF A TOOTH

uncommon. It is usually seen as a brown, hard covering of the teeth. Since it is continually accumulating, it sometimes catches on the inside of the lip, causing ulceration to the inside of the mouth.

FUNCTION OF THE TEETH

The cat's teeth are designed for grasping, tearing, self defence and grooming. There are four different types of teeth in the mouth (which is the same as dogs, and humans). At the front, between the large fangs (canines), are the tiny incisors, six in each jaw. These are used in grooming and for nibbling. The fangs or canines are the largest single rooted teeth in the mouth, and they are used for holding and tearing. They are important since they are often damaged in fights, falls or traffic accidents etc. Cheek teeth, consisting of molars and premolars, are used

for tearing and cutting. Therefore the molars and premolars, in the upper and lower jaw, do not meet (like ours), but act with a scissor action. The lower jaw of the cat does not have any lateral movement and the lower jaw (mandible) is fixed to the upper jaw via a hinge joint. This is the temporo-mandibular joint (TMJ). Therefore, cats cannot chew as we do.

The TMJ can often be damaged as a result of falls, road accidents or fights. Damage usually involves other fractures of the jaw bone or dislocation of the TMJ.

FAULTY BITES

I think we are all very aware that cats are very much more 'cat shaped' than dogs are 'dog shaped', but despite this general feline conformation, variations in "bite" do occur, particularly in association with the shape of the

head. The brachycephalic or flat-faced breeds, such as the Persian, are frequently undershot, i.e. the lower jaw extends beyond the upper. Less frequently, cats can have overshot bites where the mandibles are foreshortened. This is also called parrot mouth. Probably more serious in some of the more flat-faced (typey) breeds is the twisted lower jaw, so called 'wry mouth.'

Signs: Although faults as far as showing is concerned, these bite abnormalities do have other implications. If the cat is very undershot, the lower canine (fang) can impinge on the upper lip, causing painful ulcers. If the reverse occurs – and the upper jaw is too long (undershot) – those same lower canines will pierce the hard palate (roof of the mouth), which is equally painful!

Treatment: Modern feline orthodontic techniques,

FAULTY BITES

Normal
(incisors
level)
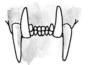

Overshot
(mandibular
brachygnathism)
Lower incisors
overlap

Undershot
(brachycephalic)
Upper incisors
overlap

Twisted lower jaw
(wry mouth)

including reducing the length of the canine causing the problem, relieves the pain of these conditions.

BAD BREATH AND HALITOSIS

Bad breath is never normal in a cat. In by far of the majority of cases it indicates dental or gum problems.

The gums and lining of the mouth should be a healthy pink colour. If the gums are reddened with inflammation, this starts as a red line where the tooth meets the gum. This is called **marginal gingivitis**. If it worsens, the whole gum become inflamed, so consult your vet as soon as possible if you are worried.
Treatment: Treatment usually involves a general anaesthetic, a dental scale and polish, and sometimes a change of diet to reduce tartar formation, plus treatment for infection.

PERIODONTAL DISEASE

This is defined as a condition affecting all the structures surrounding the teeth, not only the gums but the periodontal ligament (which holds the tooth in the socket in the jaw bone) and also the bone itself. It is the most common dental condition of the cat. In addition, there are two other conditions that occur not uncommonly in our cats, so-called **"neck" lesions** and **chronic gingivitis/stomatitis**.

NECK LESION

This is the name given to damage to that part of the tooth where it emerges from the gum. This is the 'neck' of the tooth. The condition has a variety of names, including **feline tooth decay** and **cat caries**. Interestingly, it was

only in the latter part of the 1970s that the condition was first recognised. Today, it is relatively common, recent surveys showing an incidence in up to 65 per cent of cats examined.

As a result of the condition, the tooth is eaten away (digested) by special cells called osteoclasts,

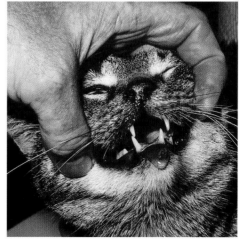
Serious malocclusion.

51

PART II

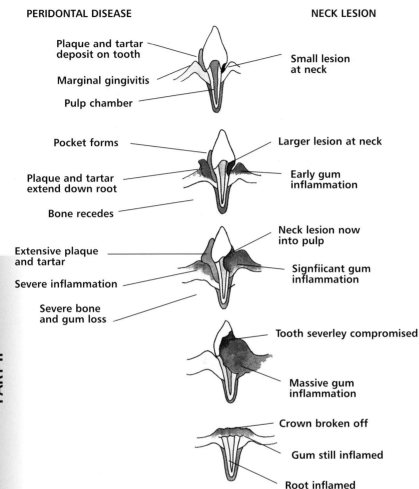

PERIDONTAL DISEASE

- Plaque and tartar deposit on tooth
- Marginal gingivitis
- Pulp chamber

- Pocket forms
- Plaque and tartar extend down root
- Bone recedes

- Extensive plaque and tartar
- Severe inflammation
- Severe bone and gum loss

NECK LESION

- Small lesion at neck

- Larger lesion at neck
- Early gum inflammation

- Neck lesion now into pulp
- Signfiicant gum inflammation

- Tooth severley compromised
- Massive gum inflammation

- Crown broken off
- Gum still inflamed
- Root inflamed

CHRONIC GINGIVITIS/STOMATITIS

This is the second most commonly seen dental condition after periodontal disease, with which it is often intimately linked. Also known as **lymphoplasmocytic stomatis (LPS)**, it affects gum tissues and often the mucous membranes lining the mouth and throat. It can be extremely difficult to treat and can affect cats from a very young age. Certain breeds of pedigree cats appear to be more susceptible, particularly Abyssinians, Siamese, and some longhair (Persian) types.

Again, the precise cause is unknown, but recent work has shown that gingivitis/stomatitis is the most reported sign in cats suffering from **feline immunodeficiency virus (FIV)**.

LPS-affected cats are also frequently found to be positive for **feline calicivirus (FCV)**, one of the viruses commonly associated with cat flu. Further, we know that when a cat is carrying both FIV and FCV, chronic stomatitis (LPS) is likely to be much worse.

It can affect cats of all ages, and in a mild form is often seen in young kittens when presented for their first inoculation. This is particularly so in breeds such as the Abyssinian and some longhairs (Persians). They will frequently be seen to have a very sore mouth and inflamed gums, which is often put down to teething. Once teething is completed around six months of age, the condition often

which are found normally within the body. Why these cells suddenly attack the teeth of our cats we do not understand at present. It is mainly in our domestic cats that this condition occurs. Neck lesions rarely occur in wild or feral cats. They are, without doubt, intensely painful for the poor cat.

Early neck lesions can be identified as small, pink marks near the gum. If you notice one, a trip to the vet is indicated without delay. They are intensely painful. Do not attempt to probe them either with your finger nail or anything else!

TREATMENT

Treatment usually involves extraction of the affected teeth under a general anaesthetic since it has been found that filling the cavity only gives temporary relief from this painful problem.

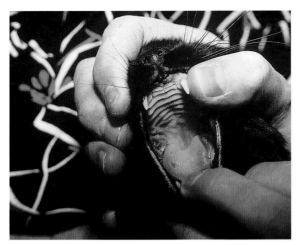

Chronic gingivitis (right internal angle of the jaw – internal commissure).

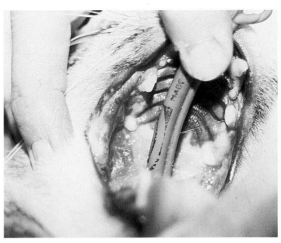

Extensive gingivitis affecting the whole of the right upper gum. (The cat is under general anaesthetic with an endotracheal tube in place.)

disappears but will usually return later in life as typical LPS.

One of the main contributing factors has been found to be the cat's intolerance to dental plaque. Plaque consists of food debris and bacteria plus certain proteins found in the saliva. It, unlike tartar (see below) is normally invisible unless special disclosing solutions are used. In the natural habitat, the plaque is normally cleaned from the teeth when a cat eats its prey. In the normal domestic situation – particularly when fed solely a commercial canned diet – plaque tends to increase rapidly, particularly the bacterial component. This is often completely harmless initially, but soon changes to pathogenic, (disease producing) germs, which quickly exacerbate the problem.

Signs: In many cats, the distinction between LPS and periodontal disease is very blurred. Typical signs are redness and soreness of the gums and lining of the mouth, often with ulceration of the angle of the jaws (internal commissures) and roof of the mouth. In young cats, gum proliferation is seen; in older cats, gum recession and typical signs of periodontal disease are evident.

Treatment: The provision of at least some food requiring effort to consume does help to control the problem. Therefore, dried food, or some of the specially prepared 'chews', can help, as does home dental care and the feeding of raw "natural" food.

DENTAL CARE

My experience – both with my own and clients' cats – is that teeth cleaning has to be started at a very early age if it is to be tolerated at all, and even then many kittens will not accept the process. Statistics, however, show that even if the cat's teeth are only cleaned once a week there is a 76 per cent reduction in plaque, whereas cleaning on a daily basis ensures that well over 90 per cent of plaque is removed. Therefore, it is worth persevering if you can.

If dental plaque is allowed to develop unhindered, it will quickly become replaced by tartar, which is a hard, brownish deposit covering the teeth. This acts as a further breeding ground for infection. By pressing on the gum, it can also cause gum recession, thus allowing further infection, with the ultimate loosening and loss of teeth.

If your cat does not allow daily or even weekly brushing routine, what can be done? Even if you cannot accustom your kitten to brushing from day one, ensure you can open the mouth so that you can regularly inspect the gums and teeth. Most cats will not object to this, particularly if they realise the procedure may be followed by a delicious treat. Some of these today are specially formulated to help with oral hygiene.

Discuss specific products with your vet. If conditions are caught early, they can be very successfully controlled if not cured. Most vets today also advocate bi-annual dental check-ups, just like us. Sometimes this may need to be followed by dental scaling or polishing, which, with the cat, involves a general anaesthetic. Nevertheless, such procedures really do help to keep chronic dental problems at bay, although, as we have seen, regular brushing – even if only once a week – really is the most effective preventative.

OTHER COMMON PROBLEMS

FACIAL ABSCESSES

These are not uncommon in cats. The usual cause is cracked or otherwise infected teeth. Not far behind are abscesses as a result of fighting. Tumours are much less common, but can take the form of a facial swelling if they are affecting the mouth or jaw.
Signs: The first sign of an abscess is usually a painful swelling,

TONGUE PROBLEMS

Cats, particularly kittens, will often play with a piece of thread or a rubber band which can get caught around the tongue and teeth. Pieces of bone can also get stuck at the back of the mouth, between the teeth, and sometimes pierce the tongue. Needles with thread are a particular danger – never leave any lying around if you keep a cat!
Signs: Irrespective of the cause, the usual result of a tongue injury is salivation, frantic pawing at the mouth and obvious distress, usually with difficulty in eating.
Treatment: This clearly depends on veterinary diagnosis. Usually a general anaesthetic will be required for examination, but foreign bodies (pieces of bone, thread, rubber bands etc.) will be removed. As mentioned previously, sometimes intensive care is required to support the cat until eating and drinking is resumed.

which may burst, releasing a quantity of evil-smelling pus. Treatment will obviously depend on accurate diagnosis, thus a visit to the vet is essential.
Treatment: If the swelling is due to an infected tooth, the vet will probably advise extraction, and often pus can be drained via the socket, avoiding the abscess having to be lanced. If, on the other hand, the abscess is not the result of a dental problem, the vet will probably lance, drain and clean the abscess, and prescribe antibiotics.

DIFFICULTY IN EATING (DYSPHAGIA)

Dysphagia strictly describes difficulty in swallowing, but the most common cause in the cat is dental disease. It can be chronic and come on slowly, as in the case of tartar build-up with concomitant periodontal disease, or develop rapidly (acute onset), as in the case of a loose or broken tooth. Other causes include injury to the jaw as a result of a traffic accident, kick, fall or other injury.

You may notice your cat is suddenly eating oddly, perhaps just on one side. Another sign is that the cat suddenly spits, hisses, backs off or runs away, although it obviously is hungry.

Salivation can sometimes be associated with difficulty in eating. Unlike dogs – some of which are naturally drooly (e.g Bulldogs) – cats do not normally drip saliva (though many cats dribble with happiness when milk-treading – anticipating mother's milk). If observed, it can be due to a loose tooth or advanced dental disease, or the result of a mouth injury or tumour. Handling to establish the cause is strongly resented.
Treatment: A trip to the vet is urgent since treatment will depend on accurate diagnosis, usually involving general anaesthesia. Once the cause of the problem has been established, your vet will advise on suitable treatment.

PART II

THE DIGESTIVE SYSTEM

Chapter 12

Most of us think digestion begins in the stomach, but it really starts in the mouth. The cat's teeth are designed to tear and cut meat into sizes that can be swallowed with the help of saliva secreted in the mouth. Cats are not able to chew their food. Saliva contains small quantities of ptyalin, a starch-digesting enzyme, but this is of little importance to the cat, a carnivore depending principally on the digestion of protein and fats.

MOUTH PROBLEMS

Digestive problems can occur in the mouth. Pieces of bone, string from a joint of meat, even blades of grass do get stuck in the mouth and pharynx (see page 49). Grass can also be coughed and sneezed back into the nasal passages, where it may lodge, causing infection.

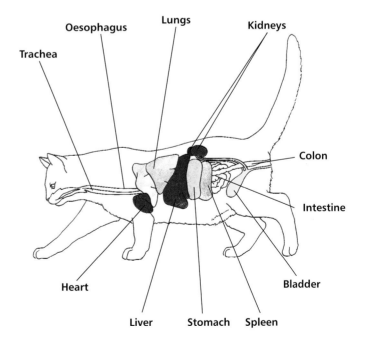

THE INTERNAL ORGANS

THE DIGESTIVE TRACT

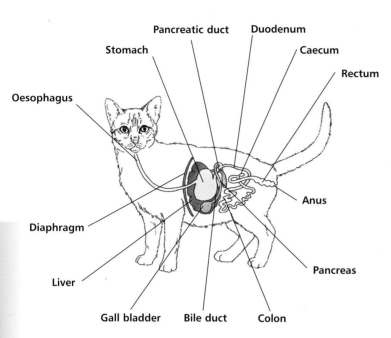

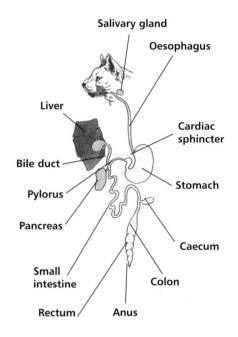

Mouth ulcers are relatively common in the cat due to viruses, (e.g. flu), general infections, and also as a result of kidney disease (see page 75).

Cats are very much more fastidious than dogs and seldom deliberately lick toxic or corrosive substances. However, they will sometimes walk in paint, creosote and other substances and attempt to lick themselves clean, causing damage to the delicate mucous membrane of the mouth and tongue.

It should be remembered that in their natural state cats frequently chew grass and other green-stuff to supplement their mainly meat diet. Our house cats will do exactly the same thing to cherished pot plants, so care should be taken in selection. Many plants contain potentially poisonous substances. Surprisingly, in view of their fastidious nature, cats seem drawn to certain types of 'poisonous' plants, such as Dieffenbachia or Poinsettia, which are often kept as houseplants.

Signs: Usually profuse salivation and reluctance to let anyone near the mouth.

CONDITIONS AFFECTING THE TONGUE

Tumours of the tongue and the tissues beneath it do occur. The signs are exactly the same as when there is a foreign body stuck in the mouth – difficulty in eating, dribbling, and pawing at the mouth – although with a tumour, the signs are usually slow in onset.

A 'burnt' or scalded tongue and mouth can occur due to hungry cats and kittens stealing or being given food at too high a temperature. If extensive, it can present a major nursing problem to ensure adequate nourishment while the sores heal.

RODENT ULCER (EOSINOPHILIC GRANULOMA)

The so-called rodent ulcer (eosinphilic granuloma) is a not uncommon condition affecting the upper lip and sometimes the nose (page 48). Veterinary advice should always be sought, since, if this spreads, it can prevent the cat from eating properly.

FACIAL INJURIES

Injuries as a result of traffic accidents and so-called 'high rise syndrome', i.e. falls from upper windows, can result in serious damage to the lower jaw and hard palate. Luckily, with today's orthopaedic techniques, the majority can usually be repaired. However, careful and attentive nursing will be required. Most cats make spectacular recoveries, provided there have not been severe injuries to the facial nerves.

LARYNX AND OESOPHAGUS

Nasal and pharyngeal polyps have already been mentioned (see page 41). Although usually benign, they slowly enlarge and can ultimate interfere with swallowing. Surgical removal is usually curative, although they can re-occur.

Problems with the oesophagus (gullet) are not as common in cats as with dogs. The usual sign is retching and regurgitation. Regurgitation occurs when food is brought up undigested, i.e. when it has not entered the stomach, or only been in there a very short time. The most common reason for this is narrowing of the oesophagus due to scarring, resulting from an injury from a foreign body, such as a lodged bone. This is always a risk – even if the bone has been successfully removed by a vet.

Occasionally, congenital heart and chest defects will also result

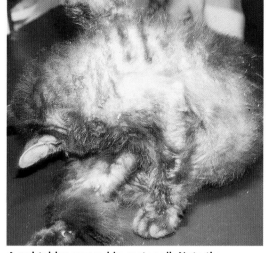

A red tabby covered in motor oil. Note the obsessive self-grooming, which leads to poisoning.

in stricture (narrowing) of the gullet. Sometimes, if there is a stricture lower down at the entrance to the stomach (cardiac sphincter), the oesophagus gradually enlarges. This condition is referred to as megaoesophagus. These conditions are rare.

STOMACH AND SMALL INTESTINE

Gastritis – inflammation of the stomach – does occur, although less commonly than in the dog. Vomiting is usually the first sign, although this can be due to many other things, ranging from kidney problems to worms, hairballs to grass eating! It can, therefore, be difficult on occasions to decide whether any action needs to be taken. For example, vomiting due to kidney problems, or worms, is an early sign needing action, whereas vomiting hairballs and grass is less important, provided it

is not too frequent.

In most people's minds, acute vomiting – when accompanied with diarrhoea – indicates an infectious cause, although gastro enteritis (inflammation of the stomach and intestine) can be due to foreign bodies, drugs etc. However, the most common cause is infection with bacteria or viruses.

Feline infectious enteritis (FIE) is the most common viral cause. Once very common, this killer disease in well-cared-for pet cats, on both sides of the Atlantic, is now quite rare due to the widespread use of feline vaccines. However, the disease is still rife in some countries.

It is very contagious, and affects virtually all members of the cat family, including lions, tigers and cheetahs. It causes very sudden vomiting and profuse, often blood-stained, watery diarrhoea. Today, in Britain, it will be seen in poorly-reared rescue kittens and feral colonies. Affected cats can dehydrate rapidly and, even with intensive care, the condition can be fatal.

Other viruses also cause enteritis – **Feline leukaemia virus (FeLV)** and **feline immunodeficiency virus (FIV)** (feline aids) are but two of these. The place of FIE in young kittens now appears to have been replaced by FCoV (feline coronavirus), particularly in cattery situations. It is seldom fatal but can be very debilitating, and it can take two or three weeks before the cat is better. The condition can

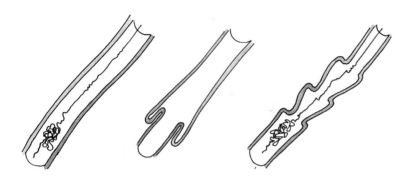

A foreign body in the intestine may cause a blockage. This can cause intersussception – when one piece of bowel telescopes into another.

be controlled with vaccination in some parts of the world.

Bacterial gastro enteritis usually causes a profuse long lasting diarrhoea. It can be caused by coliforms, salmonella and campylobacter species. Sometimes the same bacteria can cause diarrhoea in people, particularly children, and therefore veterinary attention should be sought without delay if your cat shows signs of chronic or recurrent diarrhoea.

FOREIGN BODIES
Digestive problems due to foreign objects in the stomach – or first part of the small intestine – should not be forgotten. These can be bones, needles (often with the thread attached), and sometimes hairballs. Linear foreign bodies, such as string, wool or cotton thread, may be eaten by cats. If thread is attached to a needle, it can get caught in the stomach or first part of the small intestine. The thread is pulled

along due to peristalsis (movement of the bowel), so that the bowel gets squashed together like a concertina. This is a particularly urgent problem and is very painful for the cat. X-rays and surgery are often necessary to alleviate the problem.

INTERSUSSCEPTION
In young cats with diarrhoea, one piece of bowel can sometimes telescope into another, causing a condition known as intersussception.
Signs: Signs are vomiting and usually an inability to pass faeces, although the cat strains to do so. This is a condition requiring urgent veterinary attention.

OTHER PROBLEMS
Tumours can occur in the bowel of older cats, and are often accompanied with straining (often with blood), weight loss and general debility.

Diet can cause diarrhoea, although this is not common in

cats. Dietary allergies occur, but these usually manifest themselves more commonly as skin problems, e.g. eczema, rather than bowel problems (diarrhoea). The major food manufacturers today produce hypo-allergenic diets to help this problem, but these are usually on prescription. In all cases, discussion with your veterinary surgeon regarding the use of such diets is advised.

WORMS AND OTHER BOWEL PARASITES
(see page 20, Endoparasites)
Due to the widespread use of modern, extremely effective worming preparations both in Britain and the United States, digestive problems due to endoparasites are no longer as common as 20 or 30 years ago. Regular worming with a suitable agent is advisable for all cats. Advice should be sought from your own vet, who will have local knowledge regarding the most common endoparasites in the area.

Sometimes single cell parasites, such as *Giardia* and *Cryptosporidia*, cause chronic intermittent diarrhoea in infected individuals.

INFLAMMATORY BOWEL DISEASE
Inflammatory bowel disease (IBD) due to an immune-mediated problem is recognised in cats. Often there is intermittent chronic vomiting, and diarrhoea with weight loss. Diagnosis can be difficult and may be by elimination of more obvious causes. Bowel biopsy under

general anaesthetic is often necessary. This will also rule out cancer, which can cause similar signs.

Treatment: This can be as difficult as diagnosis. Immunosuppressant drugs, particularly corticosteroids, hypo-allergenic diets and antibiotics, are the usual lines of treatment. This often has to be continued for a long time.

Other causes of small bowel diarrhoea include pancreatic insufficiency due to a lack of digestive enzymes (secreted by the exocrine portion of the pancreas), and malabsorption syndrome, which occurs when the body fails to absorb the food in the bowel that has been digested. Compared with dogs, these conditions are rare in the cat.

LARGE INTESTINE

Colitis (inflammation of the large bowel) is relatively rare in cats. Therefore, diarrhoea due to a problem confined solely to the large intestine is also unusual. When colitis does occur, signs are similar to those of enteritis (small bowel inflammation) – straining, often with the passing of small quantities of blood-stained or mucus-covered, unformed faeces.

CONSTIPATION

Constipation is not uncommon in cats. Initially, the signs may be similar to diarrhoea. There are frequent attempts at defecation – often with persistent straining. The condition is also often confused, initially at least, with other common problems in the cat, e.g. cystitis (page 77) or,

more commonly, an inability to pass urine, particularly in male cats (see page 78).

Feline constipation can be caused by simple things such as a change of environment, e.g. boarding, or even a change of litter in the tray (litter pan). Other cases can be due to pain from fractures of the pelvis following a road traffic accident or fall. These, when healed, can lead to further constipation due to a narrowed pelvic canal.

Polyps, and other tumours, in the rectum and large bowel also occur. These can also cause physical narrowing of the passage, leading to constipation.

MEGACOLON

This results from stretching of the muscles of the rectum and colon and can be caused by chronic straining. It is a well-recognised and relatively common condition in the cat, requiring specialist medical treatment, or sometimes extensive surgery.

FAECAL INCONTINENCE

This condition is probably more common in cats than in dogs. It can be due to nerve damage following injury, and sometimes infection, e.g. a severe bite wound around the base of the tail causing infection around the anus with a resultant abscess and leakage of faecal material.

ANAL SACS (GLANDS)

Cats do have anal glands but they do not cause as many problems as their canine counterparts. If the anal glands do become impacted, however, veterinary attention is certainly required.

GLANDS ASSOCIATED WITH DIGESTION

The pancreas is an important gland lying in the loop of the small intestine adjacent to the duodenum. Although anatomically a single organ, it should be thought of as divided broadly into two parts:

1. The exocrine part produces a

PART II

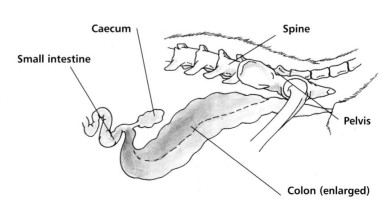

MEGACOLON AS A RESULT OF SEVERE CONSTIPATION

mixture of digestive enzymes conveyed from the pancreas to the bowel via the pancreatic duct.

2. The endocrine part consists of the islets of Langerhans, which produce insulin and other hormones. Diabetes mellitus (sugar diabetes) is due to a deficiency of insulin and is a condition not uncommon in cats.

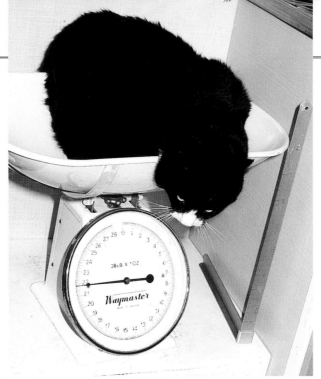

Obesity is a life-threatening condition. This cat, weighing nearly 10 kg (22 lb), is severely overweight.

Exocrine pancreatic insufficiency (EPI) is rare in the cat. Lack of pancreatic digestive enzymes causes maldigestion, with weight loss and soft, fatty faeces despite normal food intake.

The most common feline pancreatic problem is endocrine due to lack of insulin production by the islets of Langerhans. This results in diabetes mellitus (see above).

THE LIVER

This is the largest gland in the body. It is situated between the diaphragm and the stomach. As the 'chemical factory' of the body, it plays a very important role in digestion.

Jaundice is not uncommon in the cat, and is often a sign of liver dysfunction. It is usually associated with vomiting and diarrhoea, or a depressed appetite, increased thirst and general debility.

The most common cause in the cat is **Cholangio-hepatitis** (CH syndrome). This is inflammation of the bile duct and liver tissue itself, a chronic progressive disease in the cat. Causes can include bacteria ascending the bile duct from the bowel. With this type of CH, antibiotics often bring about rapid improvement.

Chronic lymphocytic cholangitis is another type of CH, but is immune mediated. Often the first signs are a swollen abdomen – dropsy (see page 71). This is more difficult to treat and often requires long term antibiotics and corticosteroids.

Chronic liver conditions often result in cirrhosis. Signs are thinness with lack of appetite and/or jaundice. Treatment at best is only supportive.

Tumours may also occur in the liver.

Signs: One of the main functions of the liver is to process waste products. Liver failure allows these toxins to build up. As a result, the cat can show signs of depression with salivation and vomiting. Liver dysfunction can result in behavioural change and, ultimately, convulsions as the toxins affect the brain.

OBESITY

It would be wrong to leave the subject of digestive problems without mentioning obesity. Just as with people, obesity in pets is now a major problem, both in the UK and US. If your cat is growing plump, now is the time to act. Get professional advice. A little help now can prolong life!

MUSCLES, BONES AND MOVEMENT

13 Chapter

Bones, joints, tendons, ligaments and muscles all make up the locomotor or 'movement' system. Major problems with any of these components can be seriously detrimental to the welfare of the cat, who is renowned as a precise mover.

Together the bones form a rigid skeleton, first to protect the internal organs and also to provide attachment for the muscles. Generally it can be said that lameness and locomotor problems in cats are often due to problems with the bones and joints or injuries to the tendons and muscles, or both, particularly when there has been a traumatic cause.

BONE PROBLEMS

Once the skeleton is formed, most people without medical knowledge tend to think that is the end of bone growth. For example, when the thigh bone has reached its ultimate size, there is no further growth. However, this is far from the truth. Bone is living and throughout life it is continuously being resorbed and reformed. In consequence there are a number of so-called metabolic diseases that can have an effect on the skeleton, both during its formation and also when fully developed.

METABOLIC DISEASE

Vitamin A (retinol) is essential for development and maintenance of the skeleton. In the cat, either too little or too much vitamin A can result in serious so-called 'metabolic' diseases.

Metabolism refers to all the physical and chemical processes by which any living thing is maintained. It refers to the processes within the body, and those by which energy is made available and used by the body. Imbalance of vitamin A therefore constitutes a major metabolic problem for the cat.

HYPOVITAMINOSIS A (LACK OF RETINOL)

The shape of any living bone depends upon a fine balance between the amount of bone that is continually produced, and that which is continuously resorbed by the body. In the adult, production and resorption have to be very carefully tuned since no further increase in bone size is required.

This is one of the functions of vitamin A. In the cat, the daily requirement of vitamin A is relatively high at between 1600 and 2000 units (iu). Compare this with a recommended daily intake in humans of approximately 5000 iu a day. This is basically because the cat, like the mink, is unable to convert carotene in the food into vitamin A. In consequence, all the

THE SKELETAL SYSTEM

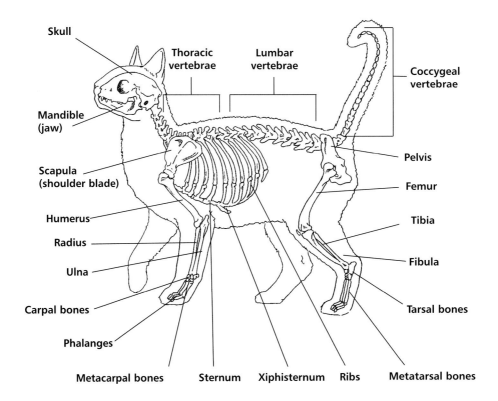

Skull
Thoracic vertebrae
Lumbar vertebrae
Coccygeal vertebrae
Mandible (jaw)
Scapula (shoulder blade)
Pelvis
Femur
Humerus
Tibia
Radius
Ulna
Fibula
Carpal bones
Tarsal bones
Phalanges
Metacarpal bones
Sternum
Xiphisternum
Ribs
Metatarsal bones

major cat food manufacturers today ensure that sufficient vitamin A is present in their commercial diets. Nevertheless, it is still considered that a lack of retinol is probably more common than is recognised, particularly if the cats are fed home-produced diets.

Lack of vitamin A produces non-specific nerve problems in young cats. This is because in the growing cat, insufficient vitamin A restricts bone growth. The bones of the skull and the spine can become distorted, causing increased pressure on the developing nervous tissue contained within. It does not end there, because insufficient vitamin A can also cause distortion of the long bones and often results in limb deformities.

Signs: The signs due to misshapen limbs are fairly obvious but nervous signs are more subtle. Lameness may be due to nerve pressure from distorted bone pressing on one of the major nerves to the legs, or where the nerve exits from the spine. In advanced cases of hypovitaminosis A, not only are there locomotor problems but there is usually lack of appetite accompanied by weight loss, together with sight and hearing difficulties due to lack of brain development as a result of a constriction by the malformed skull.

Treatment: Treatment is aimed at providing a balanced diet particularly rich in vitamin A together, of course with other essential nutrients.

HYPERVITAMINOSIS A (TOO MUCH RETINOL)

This affects cats that love liver, and it is perhaps paradoxical that those so indulged with home-produced diets can suffer from an excess of vitamin A. The effects of this are just as devastating as those experienced by the cat receiving too little Retinol, to give vitamin A its correct name.

Excess of the vitamin in the cat results in increased bone formation. In contrast with hypovitaminosis A (too little retinol), hypervitaminosis A particularly affects adult cats, usually between the ages of 12 months and five years. Exostoses (bony outgrowths) develop particularly where the nerves exit from the bones of the spine. They also develop around the limb joints.

Signs: The cat becomes increasingly reluctant to move or jump, and usually has a rigid neck and stiff back. Affected cats have coats that appear unkempt because they are unable to turn around to groom themselves properly.

Treatment: Treatment involves drastic reduction in vitamin A in the diet. In other words: no liver – which sometimes can be easier said than done since, initially, a well-fed cat will refuse any liver-less diet. However, perseverance is the name of the game, and once the level of vitamin A has been reduced, many of the bony masses start to reduce in size. This will result in an obvious improvement, although, on X-ray, the bones may show that the bony outgrowths have not entirely disappeared.

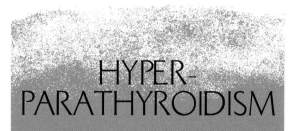

HYPER-PARATHYROIDISM

There are other metabolic conditions that can cause bone problems. Nutritional secondary hyperparathyroidism, also known as juvenile osteoporosis, occurs in kittens that receive all meat diets and little milk while they are growing. This diet results in low calcium, so the calcium to phosphorus ratio (Ca/P) is altered. This results in low blood calcium (hypocalcaemia). This stimulates the parathyroid gland, which, in turn, tries to restore circulating blood calcium by removing it from the bones.

Signs: This condition results in kittens with distorted bones, lameness due to bone pain, and sometimes spontaneous fractures.

Treatment: Treatment involves restricting exercise to avoid further injury and, of course, supplementing the diet with calcium.

RENAL SECONDARY HYPERPARATHYROIDISM

This condition, like hyperparathyroidism (see above), also results in a lack of circulating blood calcium, but this occurs in cats at the other end of the age scale, i.e. old cats with chronic kidney disease. Lack of renal function results in hyperphosphotaemia (raised blood phosphorus levels) and low blood calcium (hypocalcaemia). This low circulating calcium level again affects the parathyroids and results in bone resorption in order to release more calcium into the bloodstream.

The story is even more complicated because the kidney normally plays a part in vitamin D regulation and the condition can also result in effective vitamin D deficiency, which will prevent improvement of the condition even if calcium is added to the diet!

Signs: The usual signs of kidney disease in the old cat include excessive drinking and frequent urination. In renal secondary hyperparathyroidism, generalised stiffness and lameness are also seen. However, the most common sign is softening of the jaw bones and loosening of the teeth, thus preventing the cat from eating, so it goes hungry, which does little to help this metabolic problem. This condition is known as 'rubber jaw.'

Treatment: If the problem is diagnosed as basically due to kidney disease, treatment has to be aimed at helping the kidneys to work as effectively as possible (see page 75). A low-protein diet is recommended – as with most kidney problems – and calcium should also be provided in an easily assimilated form, usually as the gluconate or lactate, but your veterinary surgeon will advise.

Supplementation of vitamin D is also useful in many cases.

BONE CANCER

Bone tumours, osteosarcomas, are also not infrequently seen in older cats, particularly females. These are primary bone tumours, in other words, they originate in the bone. Although they can occur on any bone, it is usually the humerus (upper arm) and femur (thigh bone) that are involved. Bone cancers are very malignant, but they appear to spread to other parts of the body more slowly in cats than other animals.

Signs: Initial signs can be very variable, but often involves lameness of the affected limb, which early on can be of a transient but recurrent nature, which most owners will often put down to a bruise or some other minor injury. However, if recurrent, seek veterinary advice.

Treatment: Provided there are no obvious signs of spread on X-ray, amputation is the recommended treatment. Although drastic, it gives the cat a better quality of life since it alleviates the pain caused by the growth of the cancer on the bone.

TRAUMATIC CONDITIONS

Most feline orthopaedic conditions are due to injury, either as a result of road traffic accidents or falls. Bones most commonly affected are the thigh and shin bones (femur and tibia), pelvis and, perhaps surprisingly, the mandible or lower jaw bone. This is frequently fractured as a result of falling from a height, although sometimes if the cat has a narrow miss in a road traffic accident, the jaw hits the road with force and will be damaged.

Signs: Signs obviously depend on the bones involved. Those fractures in which the overlying skin is not damaged are sometimes difficult to distinguish from dislocations. But, in any case, if a limb is involved, the cat will not be able to use that limb.

Jaw injuries are usually obvious since, frequently, there is blood evident as a result of damage to the mouth.

Treatment: Feline bones do heal remarkably quickly, even in relatively old cats. With today's orthopaedic techniques, coupled with the advances in anaesthesia and pain control, an injury that

OSTEOMYELITIS

Bone infection is probably one of the most common problems involving a cat's skeleton. Usually it is due to bacterial infection as a result of a bite wound following a fight. However, it can follow bone and soft tissue injuries during traffic accidents, particularly in the case of so-called 'open' or 'compound' fractures where the fractured ends of the bone penetrate the soft tissues and skin. This leads to infection of the bone.

Signs: Early signs of osteomyelitis are very hard to distinguish from those of bone cancer. Intermittent lameness is the usual sign, but sometimes there is early pain and resentment at touching the limb. This is often accompanied by general systemic illness – the cat will be off-colour, disinclined to eat, and may drink more.

Treatment: Most bone infections in cats are caused by bacteria. Osteomyelitis is a serious and potentially life-threatening condition, and treatment often involves a combination of surgical drainage and antibiotics. Drains often have to be inserted into the bone, and then protected from the patient by extensive bandaging. Appropriate antibiotics, selected as a result of laboratory investigation, have to be administered, and usually also used as a solution to flush drains. In consequence, hospitalisation is necessary, and depending on the severity of the osteomyelitis, can sometimes be for weeks rather than days.

a relatively short time ago was considered hopeless is now routinely repaired.

MUSCLE AND TENDON INJURIES
Like bone problems, muscle and tendon injuries can follow fights, resulting in infection and inflammation. This is called **myositis** when the muscle is involved, and **tendonitis** when it affects the tendon. The tendon is the fibrous tissue that attaches the muscle to the bone.

Just as we suffer from torn muscles and tendons, so can cats. Ruptured tendons usually follow a sharp blow or wound. Similarly, a violent contraction of a muscle can result in tearing of either the muscle or its tendon.

Signs: Signs vary depending on the muscles or tendons involved, but, in general, there is lameness or at least significant loss of function.

Treatment: These injuries usually require surgery, and the cat often has to be closely confined for relatively long periods since tendons, in particular, are very slow healing.

JOINT PROBLEMS
Traumatic and infectious problems do not only involve bones. Joint capsules and other parts of the locomotor system can all be affected, particularly due to the cat's propensity to

JOINT SPRAINS

A sprain is said to occur when the joint exceeds its normal range of movement, and the associated ligaments and joint capsule are partially torn. Falls from trees or rooftops are often the cause. The accidents may also result in fractures of associated bones.

Treatment: Simple sprains in the cat usually respond to veterinary treatment very well, but it is important that veterinary instructions regarding restriction of exercise are strictly observed. Sometimes treatment involves confinement without any support in the form of dressing. This often depends on the cat's temperament.

defend what it considers to be its own. At least as far as bones are concerned, and, to a lesser extent, joints, cats have an advantage in that they have incredible abilities to heal.

There are a number of joint diseases that affect cats along with other animals. Traumatic injuries are by far the most common and these include sprains, strains and dislocations.

STRAINS
Cats can also suffer muscle strains, which are less serious and, in simple terms, refer to over stretching of muscles. Signs are usually lameness.

Treatment: Treatment involves confinement and painkillers. Veterinary advice is necessary,

particularly in respect of appropriate painkillers.

DISLOCATIONS
Joint dislocations also occur in the cat and are referred to more precisely as luxations. Luxations can be the result of inherited or developmental problems, but with cats, they are most commonly the result of accidents. The knee joint (stifle), hock (ankle) and carpus (wrist) are the most often affected. Slipping kneecaps (patella luxation) can occur as the result of an injury, but in certain breeds of cat this does appear to be a congenital trait that is present from birth, and may be hereditary.

Signs: It can sometimes be difficult to distinguish a joint dislocation from a fracture, even for a veterinary surgeon, without the help of X-rays. Dislocations of the joints of the limbs usually result in instability – as do fractures. The signs of patella luxation, on the other hand, are usually intermittent lameness.

Treatment: Traumatic dislocations, i.e those due to injury, require urgent veterinary attention so the joint function may be restored as soon as possible. Sometimes that is all that is necessary, but frequently further stabilisation, involving surgical orthopaedic techniques, will be required.

PART II

ARTHRITIS

Arthritis is a complex condition. The term means joint inflammation of which there are various causes, such as immune-mediated, due to infection, or the result of injury. Whatever the cause, the result will be the same – inflammation of the joint i.e. arthritis.

Degenerative joint disease (DJD) often called 'old age arthritis', is a progressive condition, leading to erosion of cartilage with new bone deposits (osteophytes) developing around the joints. Until relatively recently, it was considered rare in the cat, but modern diagnostic techniques indicate that it is just as common in elderly cats as it is in elderly people.

Signs: Just as with us, the common sign of DJD is stiffness of the joints, and in the cat, a disinclination to move.

Treatment: Modern developments with safer non-steroidal anti inflammatory drugs (NSAIDs) ensure that old age in the cat can at least be made more comfortable.

RHEUMATISM

Some forms of feline arthritis may be immune-mediated and follow a course similar to that seen with human rheumatoid arthritis (rheumatism).

Polyarthritis, where several joints are affected, can be associated with systemic lupus erythematosis (SLE). This immune-mediated disease results in multisystemic disease with skin sores, and often problems involving the nervous system, as well as arthritis affecting multiple joints. However, this condition, like virus arthritis (see below), is really very rare in the cat, particularly when compared with stiff joints due to cat bites!

Treatment: Immune-mediated arthritis in the cat can be treated but often involves long-term administration of corticosteroids and other immunosuppressant drugs.

ARTHRITIS DUE TO INFECTION

The main cause of arthritis in cats is infection as the result of bites or other joint injuries. Arthritis caused by a calicivirus has been seen in kittens as young as six weeks but this is very rare.

The take-home message has to be that if you think your cat has joint problems, see your vet sooner rather than later, particularly if you think your cat needs painkillers. Do not be tempted to relieve pain with even a quarter of one of your own favourite painkillers – you could do more harm than good.

Treatment: Treatment for the most common form of arthritis, due to bacterial infection following a bite or some other injury, involves administration of appropriate antibiotics together with analgesics obtainable from your vet.

THE CHEST AND BREATHING

14 Chapter

Feline chest problems commonly involve the respiratory system – the lungs, trachea (windpipe) and associated airways. It should be remembered that the heart and major blood vessels within the chest can also be involved.

Traumatic chest injuries are not unusual due to falls or road traffic accidents. Congenital (present from birth) abnormalities are also encountered, and in this case, it is usually the heart and major blood vessels, rather than the lungs, which are involved.

TRAUMATIC CHEST PROBLEMS

These usually involved severe crushing and bruising injuries. Despite their resilience, feline ribs can fracture, and the broken ends often cause severe lung injuries or injury to the heart or major blood vessels.

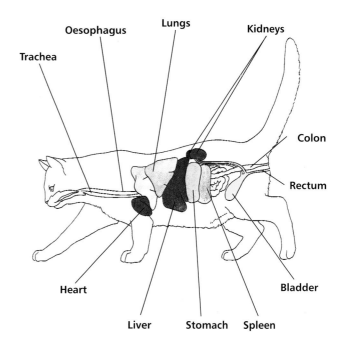

Oesophagus Lungs Kidneys

Trachea

Colon

Rectum

Heart

Bladder

Liver Stomach Spleen

THE INTERNAL ORGANS

SIGNS

Signs usually involve shallow respiration, and frequently the cat coughs up blood-stained froth.

TREATMENT

An immediate trip to the vet is essential, often for initial cardiac or respiratory support, to be followed by diagnosis, often involving X-rays and other imaging techniques. It is not uncommon for the diaphragm (the musculo-membranous partition between the chest and the abdomen) to be torn as the result of such injuries. It may have to be surgically repaired.

CONGENITAL CHEST PROBLEMS

A number of congenital (present from birth) cardiac abnormalities do occur in cats, but they are not common. They can cause sudden death in the first few months of life. If you have any concerns with your kitten regarding rate of growth or, more importantly, exercise tolerance levels, do not be afraid to consult your vet sooner rather than later.

RESPIRATORY PROBLEMS

The nose and pharynx have already been mentioned (see page 57). Foreign bodies, usually bits of grass and the occasional insect or other object, sometimes "go down the wrong way" and end up in the air passages, usually the trachea (windpipe), although

THE RESPIRATORY SYSTEM

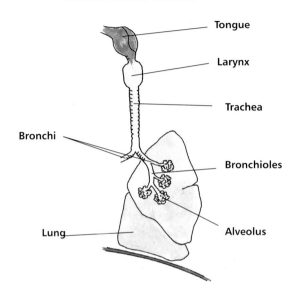

Tongue

Larynx

Trachea

Bronchi

Bronchioles

Lung

Alveolus

sometimes they can travel into the smaller airways and result in a lung abscess.

SIGNS

The first sign is usually a paroxysm of coughing. This is often successful in removing the offending object but, particularly with blades of grass, portions may be left behind.

Cats are very fond of chewing grass, especially if it has sharp blades. If any of this remains in the trachea or further down in the smaller air passages (bronchii and bronchioles), it will rapidly become a focus of infection. The cat appears off-colour with intermittent coughing, stertor (snoring or noisy breathing), and open-mouth breathing. Cats, unlike dogs, do not pant normally as an aid to heat loss. It can occur as one of the early

signs of heat stress (hyperthermia) and occasionally if the cat is stressed. For example, it occurs in some particularly nervous cats when taken to the vet. However, it is usually a sign of a severe lung problem if it persists for any length of time.

TREATMENT

Obviously this needs more than home remedies, since X-rays and other tests may be necessary to establish the exact cause of the problem. If there is a foreign body in the lungs causing infection, antibiotic treatment is necessary and sometimes surgery is indicated.

COUGHING

In general, coughing indicates a problem below the larynx, i.e. either in the trachea (windpipe) or the lungs. Pleurisy (inflammation of the membrane covering the lungs) does occur in the cat and can be the result of a chronic flu infection, but is usually associated with pyothorax (see page 69). Another cause of coughing or open-mouth breathing, and/or stertor, can be swelling due to a sting. It is not uncommon for cats to try to eat bees and wasps.

SIGNS

The swelling due to the sting is usually very obvious, involving either the mouth or throat below

FELINE ASTHMA

Prior to 1994, feline asthma was barely mentioned. Inhalant allergies were recognised, and it was pointed out that the signs were similar to human asthma or hay fever. The distinction was made that, in the case of the cat, the target tissue was the skin and not the respiratory tract, despite the fact that the allergens, pollen, dust, moulds etc. were inhaled. How things have changed in a decade or so!

In 2004, in a press release issued by the Feline Advisory Bureau, it was estimated that as many as one in a hundred cats in the UK may be affected by asthma. It is usually an allergic response with similarities to human asthma. Treatment for cats is now possible with special inhalers available. Asthma in the cat, as with us, can be a potentially life-threatening situation, resulting in difficulty in breathing due to the allergic reaction causing inflammation, swelling and constriction of the fine airways in the lungs.

Signs: Affected cats show a variety of signs, which can include coughing, stertor, general lethargy and shallow breathing. Diagnosis is not easy and involves specialised tests.

Treatment: Until recently, treatment was confined to the use of corticosteroids and antihistamines, sometimes combined with drugs to dilate the air passages. These usually had to be administered orally, which is not easy in the majority of cats – particularly when treatment is long-term.

Today the condition can sometimes be effectively controlled with long-acting injections, and relatively recently with specially formulated inhalent preparations.

the chin. A trip to the vet without delay is indicated. Coughing in any case should never be ignored. Seek advice.

TREATMENT
Antihistamines or corticosteroids administered by injection usually bring about a swift return to normal if the cough and swelling was due to an insect sting.

PYOTHORAX
Cats appear to be more prone to fluid accumulation in the chest cavity than dogs. Causes include chest cancer, heart problems, ruptured thoracic duct, or diaphragmatic hernia. However, with all these conditions, the fluid is sterile.

With pyothorax, also known as exudative pleurisy or empyema, the fluid is pus due to bacterial infection. Many species of bacteria can be responsible including *Streptococci*, *Staphylococci* and *Pasteurella* species.

The cause of the pyothorax is sometimes apparent, e.g. a penetrating wound to the chest following a fight or some other injury. Sometimes sharp objects are swallowed and pierce the throat or gullet, resulting in infection entering the thorax since cats frequently carry *Pasteurella* in their mouths.

The problem is that, in many cases, the underlying cause is just not found.

SIGNS
Increasingly difficult and shallow breathing are the usual signs. The condition is quite advanced before even the most vigilant owner notices it, and this is because cats, with their sedentary lifestyle, are experts at concealing early signs of ill health. When more advanced, mouth breathing and panting occur.

TREATMENT
Following X-rays and probably chest drainage – initially to

determine the nature of the fluid – treatment usually involves antibiotics and quite frequent chest drainage to reduce the volume of fluid and so help breathing. Since, in many cases, the underlying cause cannot be determined, some cats do not recover.

CHYLOTHORAX
Fluid from the thoracic duct – the major lymph duct in the chest – leaks into the pleural cavity. This is chylothorax. It can be due to cancer (lymphosarcoma), or damage to the duct as the result of a road traffic accident. Sometimes it follows right-sided heart failure.

SIGNS
These are the same as with pyothorax.

TREATMENT
Frequent chest drainage to reduce the fluid pressure and help breathing, together with prophylactic antibiotics, often over several weeks, until healing occurs.

CARDIAC PROBLEMS
Congenital (present from birth) heart problems are estimated to affect about 2 per cent of cats. Their severity varies. Some animals may be stillborn, others die around the time of weaning

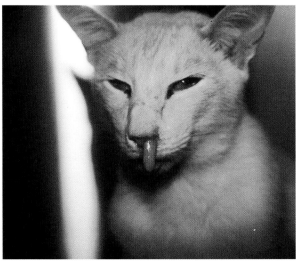

Chronic unilateral (left) septic rhinitis due to a foreign body – a blade of grass in the oropharynx.

and others show signs later in life. A significant proportion never show any signs at all, although audible abnormalities may be present when the vet listens to the heart with a stethoscope.

SIGNS
The usual signs associated with heart disease in the young cat are a failure to thrive, coupled with a poor appearance. There is usually difficulty with breathing, lack of inclination to play or to take exercise. Blueness of the mucous membranes is often a further sign, and the struggling heart is often seen to have a pronounced beat on the left chest wall.

Some of the abnormalities may be hereditary. For this reason, vets always advise not to breed from any cat once a congenital defect has been diagnosed.

COMMON HEART PROBLEMS
The most common feline heart problems are so-called atrial-ventricular malformations. This usually indicates malfunction of the valves, either on one or both sides of the heart, resulting in a back flow of the blood during ventricular contraction. As a result, the heart has to work harder in pumping the blood, which ultimately results in congestive heart failure (CHF).

SEPTAL DEFECT
This is the name given to any defect in the wall that separates the right and left ventricles. Since the left ventricle has to push the oxygenated blood around the body, if there is a hole in the wall, this blood usually flows into the right ventricle where the pressure is less. The left side of the heart thus shows reduced cardiac output, and less oxygenated blood is pumped around the body. This results in poor growth and general weakness.

STENOSIS
This refers to a narrowing, which can affect either the aorta or the pulmonary artery. The heart again has to work harder to push blood past the narrowed area, resulting in similar signs of weakness and

poor growth on the part of the cat.

PATENT DUCTUS ARTERIOSUS (PDA)

The ductus arteriosus is a foetal blood vessel that connects the pulmonary artery directly to the aorta. Within a few days of birth, this vessel normally closes so that all the blood from the right ventricle is pumped through the now-working lungs of the kitten. If the vessel fails to close, blood continues to flow from the aorta into the pulmonary circulation. This causes congestion of the lungs and overloads the right ventricle. In some cases it is possible, by surgery, to tie off the vessel and the results are little less than spectacular.

VASCULAR RING ANOMALY

This is another condition, occasionally encountered, which involves congenital defects of the major blood vessels in the chest. In the most common form, the aorta is displaced from the left to the right side of the chest. The oesophagus is then constricted between the trachea, the heart, the aorta and the now-closed ductus arteriosus.

Signs: The kitten appears normal until it starts to eat solid food when it will be noticed that, although having a normal appetite, it continually regurgitates the food. If diagnosed before there is permanent enlargement of the oesophagus, surgery, even in a iny kitten, can result in normality in just as

THE HEART AND CIRCULATORY SYSTEM

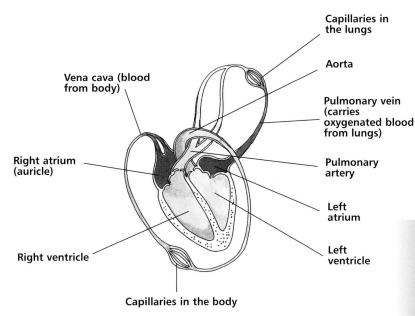

long as it takes to heal.

ACQUIRED HEART DISEASE

Surveys have shown that heart disease affects over 20 per cent of our cats. The figure may be even higher as many cats are not diagnosed because they conceal their condition for as long as possible.

Signs: The first sign is frequently the young or middle-aged cat that appears more sedentary than usual, sleeping a lot, and disinterested in playing games – usually the light from a pen torch is irresistible to most healthy adult cats. Swelling may be noticed involving the limbs or the skin around the chest. Dropsy (fluid in the abdomen), and hydrothorax (fluid within the

chest) can occur. Blue colour of all the mucous membranes (e.g. in the mouth, around the nose and eyes) is often noticed. Ultimately, as the liver enlarges due to congestion, there is often vomiting and diarrhoea.

Treatment: Today there are many cardiac drugs, which will help the heart muscle to work more efficiently and also reduce fluid retention. Your vet will advise.

CARDIOMYOPATHY

This is disease of the heart muscle.

- **Dilated cardiomyopathy:** In the 1980s, a dilated form of cardiomyopathy was relatively common. The heart became thin-walled and enlarged. It was discovered that most cases

PART II

were due to a diet deficient in an essential amino acid called taurine. Addition of this to commercial diets resulted in taurine deficient dilated cardiomyopathy (TDDC) becoming almost a thing of the past, although occasionally other forms of dilated cardiomyopathy are seen.

• **Hypertrophic cardiomyopathy:** This describes the thickening or enlargement of the cardiac muscle. This, in turn, reduces the size of the particular chamber it surrounds. The heart has to work much harder to pump the same amount of blood around the body, resulting in even more enlargement of the muscle. The heart rate also has to increase, which causes turbulence in the blood, resulting ultimately in emboli, (clots) and thus thrombo-embolic disease.

THROMBO-EMBOLIC DISEASE

Thrombosis, or clot formation, is a not infrequent sequel to heart disease in the cat. Often it is the first sign of a problem.
Signs: Tiny emboli may affect parts of the brain so that the cat develops signs similar to a stroke victim. If the lungs are affected, there can be acute breathing difficulties or, if the clot lodges in the main arteries to the hind legs, lameness or total paralysis of one or both back legs (paraplegia) can occur. The onset is so sudden that owners frequently think the cat has met with some accident, particularly since severe pain can be associated with the acute thrombosis.
Treatment: In the past many heroic attempts have been made to remove the clots causing limb paralysis, often very successfully. Unfortunately, the main cause, the primary heart problem, still remains untreated or untreatable.

OTHER CAUSES OF HEART DISEASE

This relates to heart problems arising from causes in other parts of the body.

HYPERTHYROIDISM

Due to overactive thyroid glands, **hyperthyroidism** is fairly common in cats, particularly those over six years of age.
Signs: These include hyperactivity and loss of weight, despite a ravenous appetite. The hyperactivity is usually accompanied by an increase in heart rate and hypertrophic cardiomyopathy often occurs.

HYPERTENSION

Over the last few years, high blood pressure in the cat has been recognised as a major cause of very serious heart murmurs and also eye and kidney problems.

PERICARDITIS

This is inflammation of the sac surrounding the heart. It is less common in cats than in dogs but occasionally bacterial pericarditis does occur, usually as a result of bite wounds involving the chest when infected fluid (pus) accumulating in the pericardial sac can lead to congestive heart failure.

THE KIDNEYS AND BLADDER

Cats are carnivores, which indicates they depend on a high protein diet. Digestion of protein results in toxic products, mainly urea and creatinine, which, circulating in the blood, are toxic in excess. Therefore, it is the kidneys' job to remove these, and certain other excess substances, from the body. Thus, in simple terms, the kidneys can be thought of as a highly complex, selective filtration system.

Microscopically, the paired kidneys consist of thousands of renal tubules. These are long, blind ending, convoluted tubes. The blind end is situated in the outer part (cortex) of the kidney, and is known as the glomerular capsule (Bowman's capsule). Within it nestles a knot of tiny blood vessels known as the gomerulus. The renal tubules,

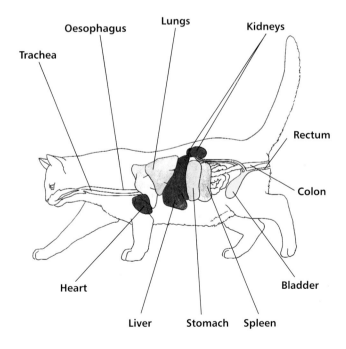

THE INTERNAL ORGANS

Oesophagus · Lungs · Kidneys · Trachea · Rectum · Colon · Heart · Liver · Stomach · Spleen · Bladder

THE URINARY SYSTEM

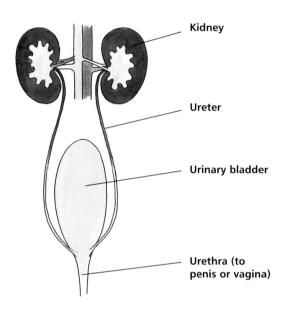

Kidney

Ureter

Urinary bladder

Urethra (to penis or vagina)

together with their associated blood vessels, pass towards the centre of the kidney – an area known as the medulla. The renal tubule, together with the glomerulus and associated blood vessels, is called a nephron. Each is a complete microscopic filtration unit. The unwanted products filter into the tubules, which unite to form collecting tubes that ultimately enter a part of the kidney, known as the renal pelvis. This, in turn, empties into the ureter – one for each kidney, left and right. Each ureter (left and right) conducts the urine into the urinary bladder, where it is stored.

When the bladder is full and the cat has an urge to urinate, the urine passes from the bladder to the outside via the urethra. This is short in the female and much longer and narrower in the male, since it passes through the penis. Urine is the final result of the kidneys' other task of maintaining the water balance of the body, i.e. volume, concentration and pH (acidity). In addition to urea and creatinine, urine also contains ions of sodium, chloride and other minerals not required by the body.

This complex filtration process depends upon adequate, but not excessive, blood pressure in the maintenance of which the kidneys are involved. The kidney also plays a part in calcium metabolism in the body, and also the production of erythropoietin – a hormone involved in the production of red blood cells in

the bone marrow.

The paired ureters, the bladder and urethra have no function apart from storage, passage and expulsion of urine to the exterior. In the male, the urethra is also used for the passage of seminal fluid formed in the testes, prostate and other glands. Problems involving this part of the urinary system are common. The cat has far more than its fair share of bladder and urethral problems, as a result of the formation of sand and gravel, which can sometimes cause blockage of the urine conduction and storage system.

Kidneys have a very large reserve of nephrons. Many cats can exist perfectly well with only one functional kidney, which is one of the reasons why kidney transplantation is feasible. The downside is that, as part of this large reserve, kidney damage, irrespective of the cause, can be fairly far advanced before there are any observable signs.

KIDNEY PROBLEMS

Irrespective of cause or severity, the first signs of kidney problems are increased thirst and increased urination – polydipsia and polyuria. Unfortunately, these signs can occur with other problems, such as diabetes mellitus (sugar diabetes), or hyperthyroidism.

As the kidney disease progresses, weight loss and an offensive breath odour are noticed. This smell is due to the increasing level of urea in the circulation and is described as uraemic breath. Due to this build-up of urea and creatinine, the cat becomes stress sensitive – even minor changes in routine can exacerbate the kidney problems, so that lack of appetite, vomiting and an increase of the uraemic breath, with accompanying mouth ulcers, become apparent.

End-stage kidney failure can result in neurological signs including twitching, head pressing and even fits. These end stages of kidney disease are known as **renal encephalopathy.**

ACUTE RENAL FAILURE

When these signs are sudden and severe, the condition is called acute renal **failure** or **acute nephritis**. Occasionally, in spite of treatment, it can be fatal but usually results in apparent, complete recovery only to be followed some time later by chronic renal failure.

CHRONIC RENAL FAILURE

Chronic nephritis involves a much slower destruction of kidney tissue. This can be because treatment, in the acute phase, arrested the rapid destruction of nephrons, but did not stop it completely. Nephron damage continued, albeit more slowly, but once more than three-quarters of the total nephrons have been destroyed, similar signs – this time due to

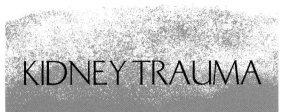

KIDNEY TRAUMA

The kidneys are particularly vulnerable to injury, especially as the result of road accidents. Chronic bruising can lead to renal failure, which often only becomes evident some time after the event. Any kidney damage as a result of injury is unlikely to heal without considerable scarring – it is the extent of this that determines the long-term outlook for the cat.

Sometimes, as the result of injury, one kidney may have to be removed. As mentioned previously, such cats are likely to do extremely well, providing the remaining kidney is fully functional.

chronic renal failure – become apparent. This usually affects middle-aged to older cats, whereas acute renal failure can occur at any age – even kittens are affected.

Kidney disease, in general, can be caused by infections, injury due to trauma, e.g. as the result of falls, road traffic accidents, etc, some types of cancer and toxic chemicals, such as ethylene glycol (see below).

DIAGNOSIS OF KIDNEY DISEASE

The diagnosis of kidney disease, no matter whether acute or chronic, is generally relatively easy. Examination of a fresh urine sample will give a good indication, which can be confirmed with blood samples, X-rays and ultrasound scans. Specific diagnosis, to pinpoint

the cause of the problem, can be extremely difficult. It may not be possible in the living animal, despite biopsies and the many sophisticated diagnostic techniques available today.

Treatment: Not surprisingly, treatment can be as complicated as the disease itself. In the acute case, the primary concern is to ensure that the cat does not dehydrate, therefore intravenous fluids are often life-saving. Antibiotics, essential in the case of renal infections, are often given together with other supportive drugs.

Treatment of chronic renal failure aims to stabilise rather than cure the condition, and is often very successful. Antibiotics, vitamins, corticosteroids, and certain anabolic steroids are often used. Diet is of prime importance. Protein intake must be restricted. Good-quality, easily digestible protein – never fed to excess – is mandatory.

Energy requirements, which, in a healthy cat are catered for by protein breakdown, can be supplied by increased fat and carbohydrates. Today there are many specially formulated diets available – the difficulty is usually in persuading the cat in renal failure to actually eat them.

PART II

CAUSES OF KIDNEY FAILURE

KIDNEY INFECTIONS

Most kidney infections are due to bacteria, although viruses can be involved.

Bacterial kidney disease may be acquired either by spread from the blood (haematogenous spread) as a result of a generalised infection, or by a so-called ascending infection when the bacteria infect the kidney via the ureters from the bladder. There are a whole collection of pathogens involved, including *Escherischia coli, Proteus, Pseudomonas* and *Staphyloccocal* species.

These pathogenic bacteria result in abscess formation. This is **pyelonephritis**. Unfortunately, early signs are hard to diagnose, but treatment with a suitable antibiotic gives a good chance of permanent cure. Otherwise the condition can progress to chronic renal failure, and it is only on post mortem examination that the cause will be found to have been recurrent abscessation.

VIRAL INFECTIONS

There are two, not uncommon feline viruses, that can cause kidney problems in the cat.

1. **Feline leukaemia virus (FeLV)** can sometimes be responsible for an immune mediated problem, **protein losing glomerular nephrophathy**. This is really a type of **glomerular nephritis** resulting in damage to the filtration units, which leads to a leak of protein into the urine, hence the descriptive name. This in turn leads to oedema, (dropsy), which is usually responsive to diuretic drugs such as frusemide.

2. **Feline coronavirus (FcoV)** is an underlying cause of feline infectious peritonitis (FIP), the "dry" form of which can affect the kidneys, resulting in chronic renal failure.

POLYCYSTIC KIDNEY DISEASE – PKD

This is an inherited condition, causing multiple fluid-filled cysts in the kidneys. It is a significant worldwide problem, particularly in Persian and Exotic breeds. It is inherited as an autosomal dominant condition, which means that every cat with the abnormal gene has clinical PKD. There are no unaffected carriers.

The Feline Advisory Bureau in the UK is doing sterling work, promoting a screening scheme in order that affected cats may be identified from 10 months onwards in order that only PKD free stock is bred.

The pressure from the cysts gradually destroys the nephrons so that, ultimately, signs of chronic renal failure become apparent. For more information, see the Feline Advisory Bureau website (www.fabcats.org).

CANCER

Kidney tumours in the cat are quite rare, apart from those associated with lymphosarcoma. This is often associated with FeLV infection (see page 98). For more information, see the Feline Advisory Bureau website (www.fabcats.org).

TOXIC OR CHEMICAL CAUSES

Renal damage can also be the result of toxic chemicals:

1. **Ethylene glycol poisoning:** This is one of the main causes of feline **toxic nephrosis**, kidney poisoning, although there are others. For some reason, cats are attracted to the sweet taste of ethylene glycol, which is one of the main constituents of antifreeze in car radiators. There is not a specific test available for ethylene glycol, but one of the effects of ingestion is the production of oxalate crystals in the urine. These can easily be recognised under the microscope. In addition, there is often a history of access to antifreeze. The take-home message is – never leave open containers of antifreeze where your cat has access.

   Signs: Signs of poisoning depend on the amount of antifreeze absorbed. Acute renal failure sometimes occurs in hours. If in doubt, consult your vet.

   Treatment: This is urgent. Intravenous fluids can limit kidney damage and hence chronic renal failure.

2. **Other toxic chemicals:** These include some antibiotics and other drugs used for treatment, e.g. Gentomycin, Amphoteracin B and

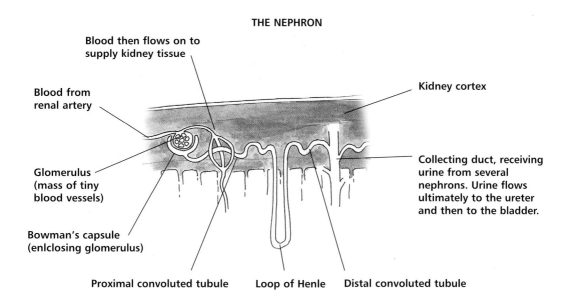

THE NEPHRON

Blood then flows on to supply kidney tissue

Blood from renal artery

Kidney cortex

Glomerulus (mass of tiny blood vessels)

Collecting duct, receiving urine from several nephrons. Urine flows ultimately to the ureter and then to the bladder.

Bowman's capsule (enlclosing glomerulus)

Proximal convoluted tubule   Loop of Henle   Distal convoluted tubule

Doxorubicin (used for certain cancers). Gentamycin and Anphotericin B are usually only used in topical preparations, i.e. applied externally, but should not be used in cats.

GLOMERULAR NEPHRITIS
Damage to the filtration units, the glomeruli, results in a leak of protein molecules into the urine, causing protein losing nephropathy (PLN).
Signs: This causes oedema (dropsy). Usually the limbs and abdomen are affected.
Treatment: Diuretics, e.g. frusemide, antibiotics and a high-quality protein diet are indicated. Eggs are ideal if the cat will eat them.

CONDITIONS AFFECTING THE URINARY SYSTEM
Moving down the urinary system, the **ureters** seldom cause problems. Kidney stones, (renoliths or renal uroliths) will occasionally become lodged in the ureter and can, if not relieved quickly, result in a swollen kidney. (hydronephrosis) and loss of function. Following trauma, particularly road traffic accidents, a ureter can be ruptured with consequent leakage of urine into the peritoneal cavity, causing potential life-threatening uraemia.
Signs: These are those of acute renal failure (see page 75).
Treatment: Treatment often involves removal of the damaged ureter and associated kidney.

URINARY INCONTINENCE
Dribbling urine is a distressing condition for both owners and the cat. In kittens it can be due to ectopic ureters, a rare congenital condition in which the ureters do not empty into the bladder but instead enter the urethra or, in a female kitten, the vagina. One or both ureters can be involved.

Surgery can sometimes be attempted to reposition the ureters into the bladder, but success cannot be guaranteed since the kittens are often frail.

BLADDER PROBLEMS
The urinary bladder, because of its size (particularly when filled with urine), is very vulnerable to trauma. It can also be affected by inflammation (cystitis) and the development of stones (uroliths).

Tumours of the bladder do occur but are relatively rare in the cat

Cystitis and bladder stones

are, together, the two most important components of feline lower urinary tract disease (FLUTD).

FELINE LOWER URINARY TRACT DISEASE (FLUTD)

FLUTD is also known as feline urological syndrome (FUS), urolithiasis and "blocked cat syndrome."

The terms cover everything from mild cystitis to total inability to pass urine. The acute form is not uncommon in male cats. This is principally due to the much longer, very narrow urethra in the male cat.

Causes include bacterial infection and urolithiasis (i.e. stones and gravel). These form either in the bladder or the kidneys, and cause inflammation to the bladder (cystitis) and sometimes total obstruction of the urethra.

Signs: Signs are usually increased frequency with pain on urination, straining and often blood in any urine that is passed (haematuria). If no specific cause can be determined, the condition is called **idiopathic cystitis.**

In many cats, particularly neutered males, there appears to be an association between recurrent cystitis and the presence of **struvite**. This is a mixture of magnesium ammonium phosphate and organic matter, which forms plugs in the urethra, resulting in straining. If the cat is able to pass urine, the increased pressure in the bladder, due to the effort, leads to chronic inflammation (cystitis).

Initially, cats with urolithiasis appear well and unaffected, apart from frequent, often painful, attempts at urination.

Diagnosis: This depends on urine examination, X-rays, and ultrasound scans etc. Antibiotics, special diets plus increased fluid intake, will reduce struvite formation.

If not controlled, this condition can lead to obstructive urinary tract disease.

Treatment: Treatment with antibiotics and analgesics usually works initially. However, unless treatment to reduce struvite and bacterial cystitis is effectively carried out, the condition returns in a more chronic form. Special diets are often required long-term.

OBSTRUCTIVE URINARY TRACT DISEASE

This is serious and life-threatening. If the urethra is completely blocked, the cat continuously strains to pass urine. The bladder fills up to an enormous size, and the cat will often cry in pain while trying to void. The increasing pressure in the bladder travels along the ureters and results in kidney damage.

Signs: Acute kidney failure (see page 75).

Treatment: This is an urgent condition, requiring immediate veterinary assistance.

The bladder has to be emptied, the blockage relieved and imminent kidney failure treated with antibiotics and intravenous fluid therapy.

REPRODUCTIVE SYSTEM

M any pet owners would probably agree that the biggest reproductive problem with their cats is the fact that reproduction occurs at all! Therefore, I thought it appropriate to begin this section with some 'hot off the press' recent developments regarding neutering.

DEBATE OVER NEUTERING

For many years there have been very strongly held veterinary beliefs that cats of either sex should not be neutered until they are approaching six months of age. The reasons were that early neutering was more hazardous due to anaesthetic risks, and that the operation itself had adverse effects on the development of the kitten if it was not already reasonably well grown. Opinions started to shift about a decade

ago with the appearance of new, safer anaesthetic techniques, but still the long-held beliefs persisted – particularly the 'stunting' theory.

However, with the advent of new anaesthetics, first in the US and then in Britain, rescue organisations started to neuter

kittens ever earlier, so that there was no chance of them reproducing when they went to their new homes. This was deemed to be important, as forecasting the age of sexual maturity has always been a major problem. Traditionally, it was considered that most queens did

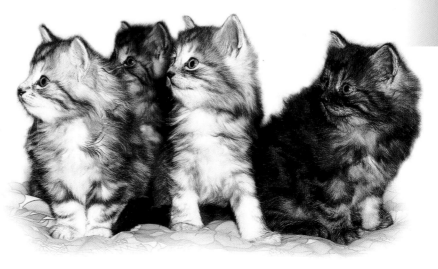

Current thinking is that kittens can be neutered at 14-16 weeks.

MALE REPRODUCTIVE SYSTEM

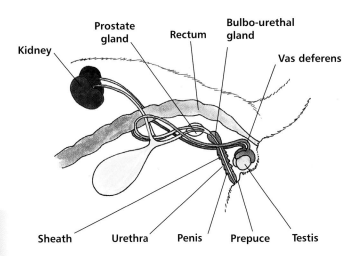

continuous during the breeding season. The queen is insatiable in her desire to find a mate throughout the spring and summer, and may well be prone to stray. To make matters worse, with central heating and artificial lighting in modern homes the breeding season is now really a year-round event.

MALES
The benefits of neutering are equally as great for males. They no longer wander and seek fights. Spraying is reduced if not totally eliminated, and even if spraying does occur, the all-pervading tom cat odour is refreshingly absent!

Having owned, exhibited and bred cats most of my life, both moggies and pure-bred, I am unequivocally in favour of breeding being left to the professional breeders. Cats' homes and rescue organisations are far too full of unwanted kittens. After a lifetime spent in dog and cat practice, I am convinced that there are few, if any, disadvantages associated with neutering both male and female cats. My view is the earlier the better; the operation is simpler, recovery is quicker and the chances of unwanted kittens that much less. Furthermore, it is cheaper, too!

DISADVANTAGES OF NEUTERING
"It destroys character," "makes them lazy", and "they run to fat," – these are but some of the disadvantages that are regularly quoted. Recent work published

not come into season (start calling) until after they were six months old, but, with better nutrition over the last two or three decades, earlier sexual maturity became the norm, so that some kittens would start to call, and become pregnant, when they were barely four months old.

The Cat Group in the UK, whose members include the RSPCA, The Animal Health Trust, The Blue Cross, The Feline Advisory Bureau, Cats Protection and the Governing Council of the Cat Fancy, as well as the European Society of Feline Medicine and the British Small Animal Veterinary Association, have recently completed a study and published figures showing that, using modern anaesthetic techniques, early neutering has few, if any, drawbacks.

Therefore, it is urged that de-sexing is worth discussing with your vet at the time when the kitten receives the primary inoculations. Neutering can then be booked for about two weeks later when the kitten is about 14-16 weeks of age and the inoculation has built up reasonable protection.

BENEFITS OF NEUTERING
Neutering does not only prevent pregnancy and the rearing of unwanted litters – there are many other benefits.

FEMALES
In the female, uterine tumours and infections are avoided, as are the problems of the "Ever-Calling Cat Syndrome." Oestrus in some breeds, e.g. Siamese and some of the other foreign shorthaired types, can become virtually

by the Cat Group, www.thecatgroup.org.uk, and FAB, www.fabcats.org, shows that obesity among pet cats can be a problem whether they are neutered or not – as anyone who regularly attends shows will know. It is my experience that, in modern society, the problem is all pervading. As far as the fat cat is concerned, careful attention to diet and exercise is required, irrespective of whether the animal is neutered or not. There are many feline diets commercially available aimed at weight reduction. Discuss any problems with your vet.

FEMALE REPRODUCTIVE SYSTEM

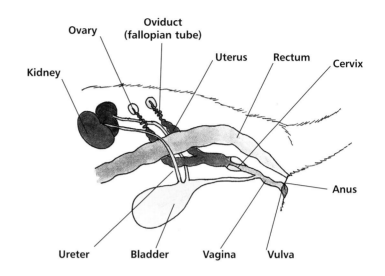

REPRODUCTIVE PROBLEMS

PYOMETRA

A frequently asked question from owners of unneutered queens is: do cats get pyometra? Pyometritis is a very common condition of the unneutered female dog. It indicates pus in the womb, and can be life-threatening. It does occur in unneutered female cats, but because of the difference in the reproductive cycles of dogs and cats involving hormone levels etc., it is far less frequent.

Signs: When pyometra does occur, the signs are very similar to those in the bitch. The queen will be off-colour, sometimes drinking more than usual (polydipsia), and she will continually lick herself due to a heavy vaginal discharge.

Treatment: The usual treatment is antibiotics and total hysterectomy.

UNDESCENDED TESTES

Male kittens should have both testicles descended into the scrotum at, or shortly after, birth. If one or both are not descended when the kitten goes to his new home, at around three months of age, the new owners should be informed. This is particularly important if the kitten is a pedigree, irrespective of whether he is intended for exhibition or simply being acquired as a pet. The Governing Council for the Cat Fancy (GCCF) regulates the majority of pedigree cat shows in this country and allows kittens to be shown in kitten classes up to nine months of age, even if both testes are not descended into the scrotum. If the kitten is being shown and approaching six months of age and you cannot find the testicles, a trip to the vet is indicated.

Treatment: Treatment is available in the form of hormone injections, but there is no guarantee you will have an entire cat at the age of nine months! However, at least with exhibition cats – unlike dogs – all is not lost. You can elect for neutering and then show the cat in neuter classes.

Neutering in these cases is really a very sensible approach since there is the possibility that the abnormality may be heritable. Therefore, even if injections induce the testes to descend from the abdomen, which is where they develop in the foetus, there is always the possibility that the cat may be passing on an inherited fault. The operation in the case of undescended testes is somewhat more complicated since one or both testes have to be located and removed from the abdomen.

FEMALE GENITAL ORGANS

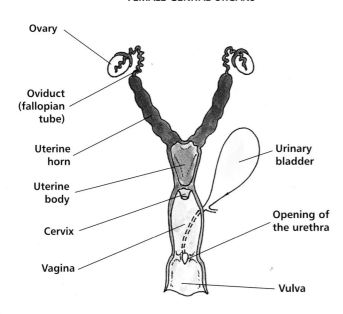

Ovary
Oviduct (fallopian tube)
Uterine horn
Uterine body
Cervix
Vagina
Urinary bladder
Opening of the urethra
Vulva

ANOESTRUS, UNSPAYED QUEENS

Similar abnormalities can occur in the female, although not so commonly. Occasionally, queens will have ovarian problems. They usually never call, although they have not been neutered. With most breeds, queens will call regularly throughout the breeding season, cycling approximately every three to four weeks. If the entire queen does not call, an operation to investigate and sterilise, if necessary, is indicated.

FADING KITTEN SYNDROME

Neonatal mortality up to 14 days after birth is classed as fading kitten syndrome. It can be due to a variety of causes. **Neonatal**

isoerythrolysis (neonatal haemolysis) is thought to play a part with some kittens. This is an immune-mediated problem whereby anti-erythrocyte antibodies are transferred in the colostrum (foremilk) from the nursing queen to the kitten. These destroy the kitten's red blood cells, due to the queen and the father having incompatible blood groups.

Signs: The kittens usually 'fade' and die within a few days of birth. All the mucous membranes – e.g. mouth, lips, tongue – appear very pale due to anaemia. Jaundice may be present with blood-stained urine and lethargy up to 48 hours after birth. It appears to occur most frequently

in longhairs and Colourpoints.

The most common cause of fading kitten syndrome, however, is **feline leukaemia virus (FeLV) infection** of the queen. Feline panleucopaenia virus (FPV/FIE) and feline immunodeficiency virus (FIV) can also play a part, as can chlamydophila infection. Feline herpes virus (FHV), no stranger to the cat due to its link with cat flu, has not been proven to be a cause of either abortion or fading kittens, although herpes virus infection in other species is known to cause these problems.

FELINE DYSTOCIA

Difficulty giving birth in the cat does not present such a huge veterinary problem as with dogs. This is probably because of the relatively uniform feline shape. With the larger cats, and the popularity of the 'flat-faced' (typey) appearance, some breeds are beginning to experience similar problems during parturition as occurs with Bulldogs, Pugs and other brachycephalic (flat-faced) breeds of dogs.

Another cause of dystocia is **obesity**, particularly in older queens. In a prolonged labour the uterus becomes exhausted and, despite careful veterinary examination, often no abnormality can be found.

Treatment: Dystocia is a serious problem, both for the queen and the kittens, and does require prompt veterinary attention. Contractions can sometimes be induced with the use of drugs such as oxytocin. A good rule of

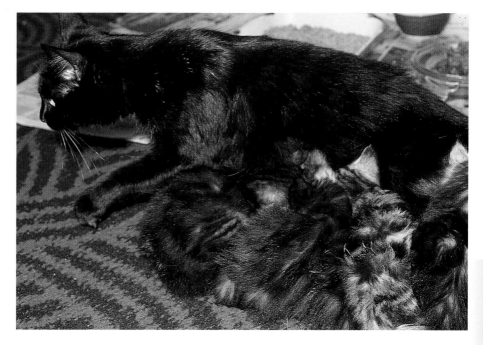

Milk fever is rare in cats, compared with dogs.

thumb is, if you have a pregnant cat that is in labour with fairly continuous straining for more than an hour without any sign of a kitten being born, contact your vet for advice.

RETAINED AFTERBIRTH

Owners are frequently worried that the cat is kittening, but no afterbirths appear to have been produced. Retained placenta (afterbirth) does occur in cats, but I have seldom found it to be a problem. In any case, cats normally eat the afterbirth as it is expelled. It is my experience that most kittening queens spend the entire birthing process either cleaning themselves or their kittens. The queen could have expelled the afterbirth – and immediately consumed it! This is

all to the good since the contained hormones aid early milk production and 'let-down'.

I am aware that many books for novice breeders emphasise the need to count the number of afterbirths produced, ensuring that they match the number of kittens. I am sure it will be a consolation to readers who have endeavoured to do this that I have repeatedly tried, but have never been successful.

MILK FEVER, LACTATIONAL TETANY OR ECLAMPSIA

This condition, much feared by dog breeders, is very rare in the cat. It can occur in late pregnancy, but more often during the first three weeks of lactation – particularly if there is a large litter. It is caused by a sudden fall in

blood calcium due to the heavy lactational demands.

Signs: The usual signs are stiffness, or difficulty in getting up and walking. Without prompt veterinary treatment it can quickly progress to muscle tremors and, in some cases, convulsions.

Treatment: This is without doubt a feline emergency. Contact your vet without delay since the queen will need special injections of calcium. You may have to hand-rear the kittens for a few days, depending on the severity.

HAND-REARING KITTENS

This sometimes has to be undertaken following a Caesarean section, as a result of lack of milk (agalactia) due to infection (mastitis), or due to eclampsia as mentioned above.

The basic needs are frequent feeding and sufficient ambient warmth. Kittens should be kept at around 32-35 degrees Centigrade (90-95 F) for the first 5-7 days, gradually reducing the temperature to 26-29 degrees Centigrade (80-85 F).

Replacement kitten food and special feeders are available commercially from veterinarians and pet outlets. Consult your vet about feeding routines, amount and frequency, even if the kittens are still with the queen. If the kittens are being totally hand-reared, i.e. away from the queen, other things have to be done, such as gently wiping around the genitals and anus with warm wet cotton wool in order to stimulate defecation and urination. If the kittens are being totally hand-reared, remember they will be deprived of antibodies contained within the mother's milk and will be more vulnerable to disease in the days and weeks following birth. Discuss any concerns with your vet. If the kittens are

LOSS OF KITTENS

Probably the most important reproductive problems are loss of kittens, and difficulty in giving birth (dystocia).

Infection: Infection is the main cause of lack of live births after normal fertilisation has occurred. Viruses, particularly feline panleucopaenia virus (FPV – also known as feline infectious entiritis, or FIE), feline enteritis (FIE), feline leukaemia virus, (FeLV), feline immunodeficiency virus (FIV) together with chlamydophila (a bacterium), all result in abortion, stillbirth or actual resorption of the foetus in utero. Sometimes the kittens are born alive, but appear weak and fade within the first few days of birth. This is popularly known as the fading kitten syndrome.

with the queen, even if she is not feeling very well, as for example following a Caesarean, she will tend to do these 'mothering' tasks instinctively.

HOW MUCH DO YOU GIVE?

Novice breeders hand-rearing for the first time are always worried regarding the amount to give, and the frequency of feeding. The importance of discussing this with your vet cannot be over-emphasised, since much depends

on whether the queen is actually contributing to the food supply, i.e. whether the kittens are getting any nourishment from the mother even though they are suckling. In addition, the breed, type and size of the kittens at birth also have to be taken into account.

A fairly rough guide is approximately 1 ml of milk replacement per kitten every 1-2 hours immediately following birth, and at least two or three feeds during the night for the next 10 days. The quantity of the feeds should be gradually increased, while decreasing the frequency. By the time the kittens' eyes open at 10-14 days, only about four or five meals should be given during the day and none between midnight and 6 a.m.

Once the eyes are open, weaning on to a canned kitten food will relieve much of the strain on the owner. The simplest way to do this is to start by mashing the canned food into some of the milk replacement and touching the kitten's mouth with a finger dipped in the mixture. They soon learn!

THE NERVES AND NERVOUS SYSTEM

Chapter 17

Neurology, the study of the nervous system and its associated problems, has always been considered one of the most difficult areas of specialisation. It is really only over the last twenty years that the cat has been considered as a separate species in relation to neurological problems. Previously, cats were automatically assumed to suffer the same nervous conditions as a dog – and not even a small one!

During the last two decades many unique feline conditions have been investigated, reinforcing my long held view that cats simply are not small dogs.

An example of this is hind leg paralysis. This is a condition that happens without warning to both dogs and cats. With dogs, the condition is most frequently due to intervertebral disc disease – a slipped disc – causing pressure on the spinal cord. In cats, although slipped discs do occur, they rarely cause hind leg paralysis, or paraplegia to give it the scientific name. The most likely cause of a cat with sudden paralysis of the hind legs is either spinal damage due to trauma in a road traffic accident, or a blood clot blocking the blood supply to one or both hind legs. In the cat, this is usually due to previously undetected heart disease. Why undetected? Because cats initially try to conceal any signs of ill health and often will have shown no detectable signs that there was anything at all the matter until paralysis suddenly strikes.

There are only a limited number of ways in which nervous tissue can react to any problem and therefore evaluation of these signs requires expertise and experience on the part of the neurologist. This applies particularly when the patient is feline, since the cat will instinctively try to hide as many of the symptoms as possible, for as long as possible!

Throughout this book, I have attempted to keep technical terms to a minimum and to define them when used. Neurology probably has more than its fair share of such terms, many of which have crept into the general language, often without clear understanding of the term. I therefore thought it worthwhile explaining the most common of these, e.g. fits and seizures, and then discussing some of the common nervous problems affecting our cats.

SEIZURES

A seizure is a fit, described as 'a physical manifestation of an abnormal electrical impulse in the brain.' Most fits last only seconds

or at most a couple of minutes.
Signs: A cat in a fit is usually conscious, on its side with eyes opened and pupils dilated. The cat may 'paddle' or appear to be running with its feet, and may urinate, defecate and salivate all at the same time. Following the seizure, there is a period of disorientation when the cat is not really with it. This is known as the post-ictal period, and can last a variable time, sometimes up to 24 hours but usually only 20 minutes to half an hour.

Since there is a post-ictal period, you are right to wonder if there is any period before a fit occurs that might give an indication of the fit about to happen. Yes, there is a pre-ictal phase, but cats, as already discussed, are skilled at hiding their symptoms, and so it is seldom noticed. It is much more definable in epileptic dogs. Observant owners will often note subtle signs just before a fit occurs. The dog will hide in strange places, sometimes appear anxious, whine and whimper. Not so cats. Few owners, even after months or years of owning an epileptic cat, feel confident about being able to detect signs that a fit is coming on.

EPILEPSY

Epilepsy is the term given to recurrent fits or seizures. Sometimes these happen so rapidly that one fit runs into another. This is called **status epilepticus**. It does occur in cats and is an emergency situation. Contact your vet without delay.

Seizures can be due to problems actually within the brain, e.g. a tumour. In this case, the cause is described as intra-cranial. Fits can also be the result of liver or kidney problems, i.e. not due to any problem within the brain itself. The fits are then described as extra-cranial. This will not be obvious from the seizure itself, which will be just as devastating to watch. It is for these reasons that it is important that a correct cause for the fits is established if at all possible. Unfortunately, this sometimes involves a number of expensive tests. In some cases, despite painstaking investigation, no cause comes to light and the condition is described as idiopathic, i.e. unknown. Idiopathic epilepsy is not unknown in the cat. Treatment, therefore, has to be directed at control of the fits since we cannot treat an unknown cause.

Diagnosis depends upon all the usual information, such as age, breed, sex of the cat, and also an accurate history from the owner.

HISTORY

This should include details of feeding and if the fits are in any way linked to a meal. This is important since, although rare, there is a condition called **porto-systemic shunt** involving the blood supply to the liver, which can be the cause of fitting in some cats. It is due to the presence of certain toxins in the blood arriving from the alimentary tract, which should have been removed by the liver,

but is not possible due to the 'by-pass' or shunt. When they reach the brain, the toxins disrupt its function and hence the seizures.

Often overlooked details, such as whether the fits occur when the cat may be stressed, i.e. visitors staying, strange animals introduced, before or after a period of boarding etc., are all important as well as details of how long the fits last.

CLINICAL EXAMINATION

A full clinical examination has to be carried out followed by a specialised neurological examination. During this, reflexes are tested. The eyes are examined not only for pupillary reflexes to light, but also for abnormalities in the blood vessels at the back of the eye. Ears are also examined and then specimens are usually taken, including blood, urine and faeces for laboratory investigation.

X-rays, including specialised techniques, such as myelography, are often essential. Myelography involves injecting special contrast agents into the spinal canal, which will show up areas of pressure on nervous tissue. If the problem is suspected as extra-cranial, ultrasound scans of organs such as the liver and the kidneys will probably be requested.

Today, much more accurate diagnosis is possible with the use of CT scans (computer-generated tomography) and MRI (magnetic resonance imaging) Clearly such investigations are expensive, but with the help of pet health insurance, full veterinary diagnostic workup, as it is termed, is possible – something that was unthinkable only a few years ago.

Unfortunately, despite all these tests, it is not unusual for no identifiable disease to be revealed. Then, as mentioned previously, the condition is called idiopathic epilepsy and we are looking at control rather than a cure.

On a positive note, idiopathic epilepsy in cats has a much lower incidence than in dogs where **idiopathic epilepsy** is a very common cause of seizures.

COMMON FELINE NEUROLOGICAL PROBLEMS

ATAXIA
Wobbly gait is a sign of many nervous diseases and can occur following a seizure, when it is usually transient. More permanent ataxia can be the result of problems with various parts of the brain. The effects of feline enteritis virus on unborn kittens is one of these (see page 96). The ataxia becomes evident as soon as the kitten starts to walk, at around three to four weeks of age. Unfortunately, it is incurable, but if the kitten is not too badly affected, at least it will get no worse. Before the widespread use of effective feline

VESTIBULAR SYNDROME

This is another idiopathic disease of the cat, and has been referred to in the chapter on the special senses (see page 38). The vestibular system provides information about the position of the body and head in space.

Signs: Signs of vestibular syndrome include head tilt, wobbly gait (ataxia), and flicking movement of the eyes (nystagmus). It is important to establish, if possible, where the cause of the problem is centred. If it is in the brain, it may be due to a tumour or serious infection.

Treatment: Such problems are frequently not responsive to treatment. If the problem is centred in the ear (peripheral vestibular disease), a tumour is a less likely cause and the prognosis much better since surgery is more successful.

enteritis vaccines, many such kittens grew up disabled in this way but, with care, lived to a ripe old age.

PARALYSIS
Occasionally, cats will be affected by partial paralysis of all four limbs. This is called tetraparesis. The cat can still move the limbs, but only weakly. Tetraplegia (or quadriplegia) is the term used when there is total paralysis in all four limbs. The usual cause is trauma, often a road traffic accident injuring the brain or spinal cord. If the hind limbs

only are affected, the condition is called paraplegia, or paraparesis where there is just weakness and not paralysis.

Although an acute onset is usually the result of injury, both tetraplegia and paraplegia can sometimes be due to slow-growing tumours in the nervous tissue.

Treatment: Depending on the site of such tumours, sometimes they show no signs until they have grown to a size that causes pressure on the brain or spinal cord with the result that there is sudden paralysis.

Sometimes cats suffer paralysis of just one limb. If this is the fore limb, the most common cause is **brachial plexus root avulsion.** The nerves to the forelimbs arise from several spinal nerves, which come together to form a 'tangle' or plexus in the armpit (axilla). Sometimes, as the result of injury, these nerves will become torn, resulting in paralysis of the limb. Unfortunately, treatment for this condition is often unrewarding and the limb ultimately has to be amputated. The good news is that most cats are able to cope perfectly well with the loss of a front leg, provided they are not obese.

If just one hind limb is paralysed this, again, is usually

PART II

due to nerve injury. But unlike the forelimb, there may be more serious injuries: often with a fractured pelvis, a fragment of bone from which has injured the sciatic nerve.

POTASSIUM DEPLETION MYOPATHY

This is perhaps recognised more as a muscle disease rather than strictly neurological. Potassium is necessary for the nerve impulses to be recognised by the muscles, allowing them to work correctly. Sometimes the lack of potassium appears to be present from birth (congenital); it can run in families, and may be inherited. Lack of potassium due to kidney disease can also be a cause.

Signs: Affected cats show muscle weakness with a typical bent neck posture.

Treatment: Once diagnosed by clinical examination and blood tests, treatment usually involves potassium supplementation. The prognosis is usually quite good, although for most cats the

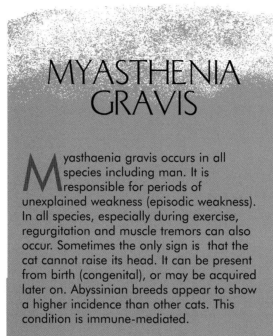

MYASTHENIA GRAVIS

Myasthaenia gravis occurs in all species including man. It is responsible for periods of unexplained weakness (episodic weakness). In all species, especially during exercise, regurgitation and muscle tremors can also occur. Sometimes the only sign is that the cat cannot raise its head. It can be present from birth (congenital), or may be acquired later on. Abyssinian breeds appear to show a higher incidence than other cats. This condition is immune-mediated.

replacement has to continue for life.

POISONING

We all consider cats particularly careful and fastidious in their habits, but nevertheless problems affecting the nervous system can occur as a result of poisoning. However, it must be said that this is seldom the direct fault of the cat except perhaps **antifreeze**

poisoning. Most cats seem to find this product particularly attractive, probably because the active ingredient – ethylene glycol – is reported to have a sweet taste! Do be particularly careful to ensure that any antifreeze in the garage is cat-proof – and that goes for products such as winter windscreen wash, which should not be left in open jugs on the garage shelf (see page 76).

Care should be taken when using anti-flea products with cats. Always read the instructions to make sure they are safe for use on cats. Do not be overzealous, since some of these products can be particularly toxic in excess. Always observe the instructions on the pack.

Signs: Over-exuberant de-fleaing can result in typical signs of toxicity with muscular stiffness, a rigid gait and sometimes excess salivation and collapse.

Treatment: Veterinary treatment is required. Certain drugs can be used as antidotes, and the cat may have to be bathed.

THE IMMUNE SYSTEM

18 Chapter

With both ourselves, and our pets, we tend to blame lack of resistance for any problems involving infections. Good immunity, although perhaps the most important, is not the only line of defence. One of the first defence systems involves the skin and the mucous membranes lining the mouth. The nose and bladder also play a major part. The liver is involved, because as the 'chemical factory of the body', one of its main purposes is the breakdown of toxins and other harmful substances that have found their way into the body.

Some of these are produced by bacteria that have invaded the body, and are broken down into less harmful substances by the liver. They are then eliminated by the kidneys. This is a similar process to that of the liver and kidneys in eliminating harmful products of digestion (see page 76).

THE SKIN AND MUCOUS MEMBRANES

The skin is a major defence organ. Intact skin prevents entry of germs and many toxins. This role is apparent when you see how quickly even minor cuts and scratches become infected if neglected.

The nasal and oral passages are largely lined with tiny hair-like structures known as cilia. These trap dust, bacteria and other harmful particles, and by their movement waft them towards the outside. Coughing and sneezing is then designed to eliminate them.

Tears, together with saliva, stomach acid and mucus in the bowel, all provide lines of resistance to trap and eliminate foreign invaders.

Without these mechanisms it is doubtful whether immunity alone would be effective.

WHAT IS THE IMMUNE SYSTEM?

The immune system broadly consists of lymph nodes together with organs such as the spleen, thymus, lung, liver and white blood cells (leucocytes).

Leucocytes are made in the bone marrow. There are several types of leucocytes each with a particular role as part of the defence mechanism of the body. Some, such as **neutrophils** and **monocytes,** are scavenger cells engulfing any bacteria or other harmful organisms, which are then killed and broken down into relatively harmless substances by enzymes released by the engulfing scavenger cells.

Neutrophils are usually the first line of defence; the monocytes arrive later once the inflammatory process is underway. Monocytes are also found within tissues when they are called **macrophages**, e.g. in lung tissue, where there are huge numbers. Air breathed into the lungs always contains variable numbers of micro-organisms that have avoided earlier lines of defence, such as cilia. The macrophages in the lungs act as a secondary line of defence ensuring, as far as possible, that further penetration into the body is prevented.

The liver is another site for macrophages. Here, their job is to engulf any harmful bacteria that have found their way into the bloodstream from the bowel during digestion.

The feline immune system can be thought of as being composed of two parts:-

1. **Non-specific immunity:** This comprises neutrophils and macrophages together with other first-line defence mechanisms, such as the skin and the cilia of the mucous membranes. Others, such as the liver and the acidic juices present in the stomach, are also 'non-specific'. This non-specific immunity kills many microorganisms taken in with food before they have a chance to reproduce and cause problems for the cat. Tears act in a similar way to protect the eyes.

2. **Specific immunity:** It is on this we depend when we employ vaccination to protect against certain diseases. Approximately 25 per cent of

the circulating white blood cells of the cat consist of lymphocytes. These tend to congregate in large numbers in those tissues associated with the production of antibodies. These include the lymph nodes, the spleen and the bone marrow. Infective agents, e.g. bacteria and viruses, are composed largely of protein molecules called antigens. Particular lymphocytes known as B-lymphocytes attach to these antigens, which causes the B-lymphocytes to divide to produce cells called plasma cells, which can produce antibodies. These are substances that can, in turn, combine with the antigen to render it harmless.

Unlike non-specific immunity, an antibody is specific for the particular antigen. This, in very simple terms, is how vaccination works.

Following an injection of a vaccine, a controlled amount of antigen is presented to the B-lymphocytes. As antibodies are produced, this protects the cat from further infectious agents carrying the same antigen.

However, that is not the end of the story. The antibody produced works in a number of ways:

- It can render inactive the bacterial toxins known as antigens.
- It can break down the bacteria, viruses or protozoan (single cell) invaders themselves.

- It can promote ingestion of the infected agent by the monocytes (macrophages).
- Antibodies can act as a trigger mechanism for other defence systems in the body.

Should this not be sufficient, the body also has a secondary line of defence. Antibody production is technically known as '**humeral response**'. In addition, there is a **cell-mediated immunity**. This acts through another, larger type of lymphocyte known as a **T-cell**. When presented with the same antigen as the B-cells, the T-cells are also sensitised to it and can recognise it on other cells and kill them. This can happen with virus-infected cells, tumour cells, etc.

Compared with non-specific immunity, it will be realised that these defence mechanisms are complex and take longer to become effective. Therefore, a detectable amount of antibody cannot normally be demonstrated in the circulation until at least five days after a particular antigen has been detected by the B and T lymphocytes. The good news is that when the same antigen or infection occurs on subsequent occasions, the cat's immune system is already on full alert and a complete response takes place in 48-72 hours. This is the basis of successful vaccination!

However, it should not be thought that this response is only as a result of vaccination. Throughout the cat's life, similar reactions are taking place on a continuous basis, with the ever-watchful lymphocytes detecting foreign antigens. Thus throughout life, the cat is building up a workable immunity against a whole range of possible life-threatening infections. Protection is passed on by the pregnant queen to her kittens, before birth via the bloodstream through the umbilicus, and after birth through the milk, particularly the rich foremilk or colostrum. This is produced for a day or two after giving birth. There are also some antibodies in the normal milk supply, and these can be absorbed during the period the kitten is suckling.

It is for this reason that it is essential that, if at all possible, kittens receive at least some colostrum shortly after birth. For the first few weeks of its life, the kitten is thus protected under the umbrella of the mother's immunity while its own immune system develops. This can sometimes be a disadvantage. For example, if vaccination of the kitten is carried out too early, the circulating maternal antibodies kill the antigens in the vaccine, and the kitten will not develop the necessary protection. Vaccine manufacturers continuously endeavour to produce vaccines that will be effective in the face of circulating maternal antibodies, and great strides have been made in the last few years, so that the first inoculations can be administered when necessary, as early as six weeks of age. This is useful, for example, for litters born in situations of high risk, such as those in rescue centres.

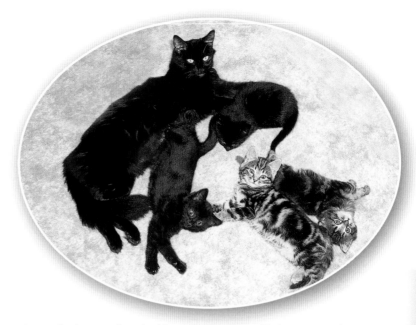

Immunity is passed to the kittens in the first milk, known as colostrum.

AUTOIMMUNE DISEASE

I hope my brief outline of the theory of immunity will, at least, go some way towards making the theory of **autoimmunity**, and in particular **autoimmune disease**, more intelligible.

Primarily, the immune system is concerned with the elimination of antigens from the body. These antigens, i.e. foreign proteins, may be bacteria, viruses, parasites etc. Similar proteins are present as part of the body's own tissues. Therefore it is important that the body recognises its own protein particles – 'self' from 'non-self'– foreign proteins (antigens). Unfortunately, this does not always happen and, occasionally, the body mounts a defence against its own proteins, which results in tissue damage. This is the basis of **autoimmune disease**.

FELINE AUTOIMMUNE DISEASE

Autoimmune problems in the cat appear, at the moment, to be less important than in some other species including ourselves. This may well be due to our present lack of knowledge of the problem in relation to the cat.

We do know that feline autoimmune disease in the cat includes **autoimmune haemolytic anaemia (AIHA), immune mediated thrombocytopaenia, (IMT)** and **systemic lupus erythematosis (SLE)**. In all of these, 'self' protein is mistaken for 'non-self' and, in attempting to eradicate it, serious damage is done to the body.

WHY DOES THIS OCCUR?

At present there are a number of theories:
• Several feline immuno-

suppressant viruses are recognised. These include FIV, FeLV and FCoV (see pages 97-99). It is thought that the immune response stimulated in some cats not only acts against the virus and the cells it is inhabiting, but also similar healthy cells.

- Cancers of the lymphoid or immune system itself can lead to the production of foreign proteins (antigens) against which the body mounts a defence. If this defence gets out of hand, not only is the cancer destroyed, but also healthy cells, and problems of autoimmune disease arise.

- Some drugs can become attached to cell proteins. These appear to the body to be an antigen, and so it develops antibodies in order to destroy it. The antigen/antibody complexes, when formed, can then disrupt the tissue. This is thought to be the reason why some drugs are nephrotoxic in the cat.

- Potentially antigenic proteins in the body, e.g. spermatozoa and lens protein are normally isolated from the immune system. Sometimes this

TREATMENT OF AUTOIMMUNE CONDITIONS

At present, treatment of all these autoimmune conditions does not carry a very good prognosis – although long-term stabilisation is achievable. Corticosteroids, in high doses, are the popular drugs of choice used to control the immune response. These, in themselves, can have side-effects and often have to be combined with much more expensive immuno-suppressant drugs, such as azothioprine, in order to achieve a reasonable quality of life for the patient.

natural barrier breaks down, and then these proteins are treated as 'foreign'.

SYSTEMIC LUPUS ERYTHEMATOSIS (SLE)

SLE is rare in the cat compared with the dog, but the signs are very similar.

Signs: There is usually arthritis involving multiple joints. Skin lesions (eczema type) often occur, affecting the junction of mucous membrane and skin. Common sites are the nostrils, the corners of the lips and the anus. The kidneys can be affected, leading to a condition called **protein losing nephropathy (PLN).** As a result, the kidney is no longer able to retain essential protein in the circulation, and its loss leads to dropsy. SLE sometimes causes destruction of blood cells, including red and white cells and also blood platelets.

GLOMERULAR NEPHRITIS

This is a serious autoimmune kidney problem and occurs when antigen/antibody complexes are deposited in the capillary walls of the kidney glomeruli (see page 77). The result is irreparable damage to these vital kidney cells. The condition in the cat is often associated with FeLV, FIP and sometimes FIV. The tremendous loss of protein leads to swelling, particularly of the limbs (oedema) and sometimes fluid in the abdomen (dropsy). Onset of signs is usually slow and insidious, but occasionally occurs very rapidly.

OTHER CONDITIONS

Other immune-mediated conditions include **autoimmune haemolytic anaemia**, a type of **progressive polyarthritis** and **myasthaenia gravis**. These are rare in the cat.

INFECTIONS

I nfections can be caused by bacteria, viruses, fungi, and also other organisms, such as protozoa – microscopic, one-celled organisms. Because the cat has an infection, e.g. a virus, it does not necessarily mean there will be signs of disease. For example, cats can often be infected with cat flu viruses and actually shed them, and, thus, act as a risk to other cats without showing any signs at all.

With cats we think of most infectious diseases being caused by either viruses (such as cat flu or feline enteritis), bacteria (e.g. *staphylococci* and *coliforms*, which often cause abscesses), or fungi (e.g. microsporum, which causes ringworm).

However, there are other organisms that can cause disease in cats, such as chlamydophila (originally chlamydia). At one time this was classed as a virus,

but has now been reclassified as a bacterium because it is susceptible to some antibiotics.

Today we depend upon antibiotics to fight most of the bacterial diseases. It should be remembered that viruses are not susceptible to antibiotics, and although effective anti-viral agents are becoming available, we still depend to a huge extent upon the body's ability to fight the virus with its own antibodies (see page 89, immune system). It is upon this that the whole concept of vaccination depends. Cats are today regularly vaccinated against a variety of virus diseases, cat flu and feline enteritis among them. The aim is to inject suitably weakened, or, in some cases, killed varieties of the causal

organism (the virus) in order that its specific proteins (called antigens) will stimulate the body to produce sufficient antibodies. These antibodies will combine with the antigens of any future, similar viruses that invade the body and thus protect the cat.

Vaccines are also available to protect against bacterial and chlamydophyial infections.

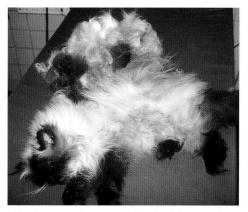

Infections can be passed from cat to cat when they are licking and grooming each other.

Chlamydophila produces flu-like disease in susceptible cat colonies.

HOW IS DISEASE SPREAD?

Transmission depends on the infectious agent involved. Diseases can be passed from one cat to another – either directly, as the result of sniffing, licking, biting etc., or indirectly when the infected cat sheds the particular agent (virus, bacteria etc.) and a susceptible cat picks it up from the ground, cage, food bowl or, for that matter, contact with the owner. Thus, prevention of infection is not always achieved by simply keeping your cat away from a sick cat.

COMMON CAT INFECTIONS

FELINE ABCESSES

Cats' mouths are well known for the number of potentially pathogenic bacteria that they contain. Therefore, it is no surprise that cat bite abscess is by far the most common infection of cats in the UK and the USA. In fact, this does not only apply to cats. If we get bitten by a cat, no matter how superficially, medical advice should be sought without delay, since a variety of disease-producing bacteria can be inoculated as a result of the bite, which can result in serious medical problems if treatment is delayed.

Often the first sign that a cat is developing an abscess is the appearance of a fluid-filled swelling, which may ultimately burst, releasing quantities of evil

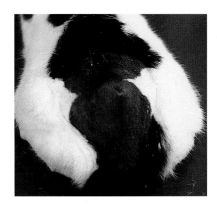

Swelling due to an abscess on the lower back, which is about to burst.

smelling pus. By that time the cat is likely to be off colour in other ways, so it is good practice to consult your vet if there is any unusual swelling on your cat. Once burst (or lanced by the vet), most abscesses usually clear up in a few days, particularly if antibiotics have also been prescribed.

In a certain number of cats, cat bite abscesses will not clear up according to plan. If the cat is not receiving any type of immunosuppressant medication, e.g. corticosteroids, the usual reason for lack of healing is the presence of one of the immunosuppressant viruses, FeLV or FIV.

Sometimes you will have no idea the cat is developing an abscess until it presents with a wound, dripping pus.

FIRST AID

Initially, bathe the area with salt water. Dissolve a level teaspoonful of salt in a large cup of water. Since cats are particularly sensitive to certain antiseptic and

disinfectant solutions, it is better not to use these unless you happen to have something that has been specifically prescribed by your vet, whereas salt water will do no harm. Then take your cat to the vet without delay.

OTHER BACTERIAL PROBLEMS

BORDETELLA INFECTION

So-called kennel cough, (**Bordetellosis**) is a well-known problem in dogs and can be caused by certain viruses and by the bacterium *Bordetella bronchiseptica* against which there has been a canine kennel cough vaccine for many years. A similar bug can cause sneezing and a sore throat in cats, and can sometimes be a problem in catteries to such an extent that feline vaccines are now commercially available to prevent the infection (*Bordetellosis*).

However, the bug involved is sensitive to antibiotics such as oxytetracycline or doxycycline, but nevertheless the vaccine is useful as a preventative in high-risk situations, such as boarding catteries, where *Bordetella* is known to occur.

CAMPYLOBACTER INFECTION

This is occasionally responsible for diarrhoea in cats as it can be in people. If there are recurrent occurrences of diarrhoea, or if you have a sick cat that suddenly develops diarrhoea, it is worth discussing this with your vet, since *Campylobacter jejuni,* the causal organism, can infect people. Scrupulous hygiene should be practised when clearing up after your cat. Always wash your hands thoroughly.

CHLAMYDOPHILA (CHLAMYDIA PSITTACI) INFECTION

At one time this was called **feline pneumonitis** and previously known as **chlamydiosis**. In cats, it can be the source of persistent conjunctivitis and can easily pass from cat to cat. Vaccines are available on both sides of the Atlantic and are useful in colonies where there is chronic infection. Runny eyes are often associated with sneezing and a runny nose, hence the name pneumonitis, although *chamydophila* seldom causes pneumonia. Antibiotics are available to treat the condition and if there are other in-contact cats these should also be treated unless, of course, they are fortunate enough to have been vaccinated.

OTHER NON-VIRAL INFECTIONS

LYME DISEASE

Borreliosis or Lyme disease is caused by a spirochete organism (which is a tightly coiled, microscopic bacterium), *Borrelia burgdorferi*. The organism is transmitted by the bites of ticks and can infect humans as well as dogs, cats and other animals. Although cases do occur in the UK, the disease is much more prevalent in the US.
Signs: In cats, the usual clinical signs are recurring lameness in one or more limbs with a raised temperature and swollen glands.

Cardiac, kydney and neurological problems have also been reported. Laboratory tests are required to confirm diagnosis. If you live in a Lyme disease area and your cat is lame during the months of tick activity, a trip to the vet is well worthwhile.
Treatment: Once a positive diagnosis has been made, antibiotics should be used as early as possible. This is why it is essential to visit your vet as soon as possible. Most broad-spectrum antibiotics are effective, but have to be used for up to one month. Vaccines are available in North America, but not in the UK. Prevention depends on preventing tick bites; the use of feline-licensed spot-on, or anti-parasite spray-on, preparations are usually effective.

Provided diagnosis is made early, antibiotic therapy is usually effective, and the cat should make a good recovery.

SALMONELLA INFECTIONS

Most people today are aware of salmonella food poisoning. Interestingly, Salmonella species of bacteria, particularly *salmonella typhimurium,* can occasionally affect cats, although they do seem to have a much higher level of natural immunity than we have. Nevertheless, cats can be affected as a result of eating infected foodstuffs, particularly from rubbish dumps etc.
Signs: Lethargy, fever, diarrhoea, vomiting and weight loss are the usual signs.
Treatment: Salmonella infection is susceptible to a number of antibiotics. The danger is that the

infected cats can shed the Salmonellae, and thus can be a hazard to any people or animals around them.

CANDIDIASIS (ORIGINALLY KNOWN AS MONILIASIS)

This is a disease that occurs occasionally in cats, caused by a yeast organism (**Candida albicans**), which normally inhabits the mouth, nose and ears without causing problems. If transmitted to other parts of the body in susceptible cats, it can be extremely serious.
Signs: The signs are very similar to feline infectious peritonitis (FIP) (see page 97) and, like this disease, is often associated with an infection of one of the immunosuppressive viruses, FeLV or FIV. The disease can occur as a chronic infection of the skin, ears and mucosal surfaces. Lesions are typically grey plaques with a foul smell.
Treatment: Veterinary treatment is essential. Antifungal drugs, e.g. nystatin, itraconazole and ketoconamole, are used, but obviously checks have to be carried out to establish whether the cat is FIV or FeLV positive.

CRYPTOCOCCOSIS

This is a common fungus infection of cats in the United States although rare in England. It can affect the skin, nose, lungs, eyes and nervous system. Infected cats become chronically ill with weight loss, lack of appetite, depression, fever, sneezing etc. Swellings may arise that initially look like cancer with polyp-like growths hanging

PART II

from the nostrils. This is a serious disease. If suspected, veterinary attention should be sought without delay.

Treatment: This involves the use of ketaconazole and other antifungal preparations.

SPOROTRICHOSIS

This is a fungal disease that does not occur in the United Kingdom although it can cause problems in the US. The causal organism, *Sporothrix spp,* lives in the soil. It can be introduced into the body by a scratch from a contaminated claw. It is communicable to humans (zoonotic), and causes multiple abscesses and a serious skin infection known as cellulitis. Cats often spread the infection by grooming. Occasionally, it affects internal organs.

Treatment: Like most of the fungal (mycotic) infections, sporotrichosis is difficult to treat, mainly because many of the antifungal preparations available are very toxic to cats. If confined to the skin, treatment with antifungal drugs and also sodium iodide is likely to be successful. If the fungus has spread internally, the prognosis is grave.

RINGWORM

Although theoretically a skin infection, ringworm is often classified as a parasitic problem (see page 20).

VIRUS DISEASES

FELINE ENTERITIS (FELINE PANLEUCOPAENIA)

Feline infectious enteritis (FIE),

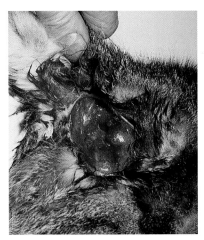

A ruptured abscess at the base of the tail.

virus or feline parvovirus (FPV) as it is now called, was the first cat virus to be isolated. It is found in all parts of the world, and until the manufacture of an effective vaccine, feline enteritis killed millions of cats worldwide. It is similar to, but not the same virus, as canine parvovirus (CPV), which causes a similar illness in dogs. Part of its success as a killer disease is its resistance. It is able to live in the environment for a long time. Today the disease is seldom seen either in the UK or the US in domestic cats. This is due to widespread vaccination. However, it remains very prevalent in the domestic cat population in many of the poorer countries of the world.

Cats are usually infected by mouth. The incubation period, which is the time between infection and showing first signs, is about 2-10 days.

Signs: Fever, depression, lack of eating (anorexia) and dehydration

occur very quickly. Sometimes the disease progresses so rapidly that the cat does not have time to show the classic signs of diarrhoea ('feline enteritis') and instead may vomit blood. In acute cases, despite supportive treatment, the cat will be dead within 2-3 days.

Treatment: As with all virus diseases, there is no specific cure at the moment. Treatment has to be supportive, ensuring that the patient is kept warm and comfortable, and dehydration is combated with provision of intravenous infusions.

CAT FLU

This is another worldwide feline disease caused mainly by either feline calicivirus (FCV) or feline herpes virus (FHV), which is also known as feline viral rhinotracheitis virus (FVR). The most serious cases of cat flu are caused by FHV. Occasionally, both viruses are involved at the same time. Unlike feline enteritis, flu viruses are not particularly hardy. FHV will only live about 24 hours away from the body, whereas FCV lasts for up to 7 days.

Spread occurs mainly in two ways:

1. Infected droplets can travel up to 2 metres when sneezed out by an infected cat, so that any susceptible cats in the proximity can be infected.
2. Direct contact either with the infected cat, or its discharges, faeces or urine, contaminated feeding bowls, litter trays and food, etc. This is known as fomite spread.

Thus, prevention of spread depends upon trying to prevent infected cats sneezing over dishes, food, etc., to be used by other cats. Scrupulous hygiene, hand washing, etc., should always be practised.

Signs: Irrespective which virus causes the disease, the first signs are usually sneezing and runny eyes. Often the cat will have a fever at first. Cats are often anorexic (off food) because they cannot smell their food. As the disease progresses, the two viruses cause slightly differing signs. FCV causes ulcers in the mouth and on the tongue so the cat will drool and be unable to eat. FHV often causes ulceration of the cornea (the clear part in the front of the eye), and can often cause chronic sinusitis or rhinitis, leading to the so-called 'snuffly cat'/'snotty cat' syndrome (see page 40).

Other infectious agents also tend to act as hangers on. Chlamydophila (see page 94) causes conjunctivitis and may be mistaken for cat flu, which is sometimes also involved. *Bordetella bronchiseptica* (see page 94) causes similar signs. In addition, one of the after-effects of flu, 'chronic snuffler syndrome' can be due to the cat being immuno-suppressed due to FeLV or FIV infection.

In the US (but not in the UK) other infections, such as *Cryptococcus, Aspergillus* and

PYOTHORAX

This means pus in the chest cavity. It is not a rare condition in the cat. There are a whole range of bacteria that can be responsible. Frequently the condition develops without signs of previous injury, such as a chest wound or bite.

Signs: The usual signs are breathing difficulties and frequently the condition is quite advanced before anything untoward is noticed.

Treatment: Treatment can involve considerable veterinary attention, including antibiotics and frequent chest drainage. In spite of treatment, in some cases the condition is fatal (see page 69).

Blastomyces, also contribute. In chronic cases of cat flu, bacteria such as *Pasteurella* will invariably be involved in chronic rhinitis (nasal infection).

Viruses can also cause other problems. FCV is associated with chronic gingivitis (gum imflammation) in otherwise healthy cats, whereas FHV in neonates (kittens only a few hours to days old), can result in 'fading kitten' syndrome, causing kittens to die within a few days. The problem is that cats infected with either FCV or FHV continue to excrete the virus even if they have recovered from clinical signs and appear healthy. FHV is shed intermittently usually following stress such as re-homing, going into boarding, kittening etc. Unfortunately, the carrier cat seldom loses the infection completely.

FCV cats, on the other hand, shed the virus continuously. The good news is that, not infrequently, cats spontaneously recover and eliminate FCV from their bodies.

Interestingly, a recent survey has shown that over 85 per cent of cats with chronic gingivitis, showing no other signs, were positive for FCV. Regretfully, vaccination, even when the cat has recovered and appears healthy, will not prevent shedding of the virus; it will certainly prevent signs of further disease, although the cat will continue to be a source of infection to susceptible cats due to virus shedding.

Treatment: Despite the fact there is no specific treatment for cat flu, as soon as the condition is suspected a trip to the vet is worthwhile, since, although the virus cannot be directly treated with drugs, the bacterial secondary invaders – which cause many of the symptoms – are susceptible to antibiotics and can be successfully eliminated, thus giving the cat a better chance to overcome the virus. Over the last two to three years, new anti-viral drugs have become available that show promise.

FELINE INFECTIOUS PERITONITIS (FIP)

This is a worrying and not uncommon condition of cats. It is caused by a virus with 'a twist in

PART II

its tail'. Feline coronavirus (FCoV) can often be detected in the intestines of the cat and most of the time is not a troublemaker, although similar viruses do occur in dogs and pigs and are responsible for definite coronavirus enteritis. In a small percentage of cats, the virus appears to leave the intestine and cause inflammation of the blood vessels, especially those in the abdomen. This vasculitis (inflammation of the blood vessels) particularly affects the vessels in the lining of the abdomen (the peritoneum), causing peritonitis (inflammation of the peritoneum), which is one of the reasons for the fluid accumulation, and hence, the slowly enlarging abdomen due to ascites (dropsy).

On occasion, vasculitis occurs in other organs, such as the liver, the kidneys, brain or eye, and in these cases fluid accumulation is absent. Instead, the vasculitis results in granuloma formation, i.e. an accumulation of inflammatory cells attempting to heal the defect in the body's defences. If this happens in the eye, or any other essential organ, the signs can be very diverse, culiminating in blindness, fits, kidney failure etc.

FIP can affect a cat of any age, although it is seen most frequently in cats under two and over nine years. Sometimes the development of peritonitis and massive abdominal fluid retention is very rapid, whereas in other cases it is slow and insidious with the cat just being a little 'off song' for a

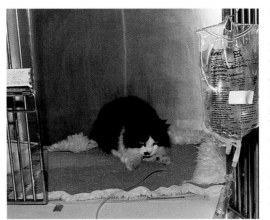

Intravenous fluid therapy is used to combat dehydration.

few months. Although heroic attempts to relieve suffering may be made by the veterinarian, e.g. repeated draining of the abdomen, unfortunately there is no cure and ultimately the cat will die, or have to be put to sleep on humane grounds.

FCoV is a very infectious virus. If suspected, a trip to the vet is necessary, if only to put your mind at rest, since there are many other causes of a swollen abdomen – pregnancy being one of them! If you have more than one cat, laboratory tests are advisable to establish whether any others are infected. Your vet will also be able to give you specialist help regarding prevention of spread to other cats. This is particularly important if breeding stock is involved.

FELINE IMMUNODEFICIENCY VIRUS (FIV)

Problems associated with this virus have been recognised in cats both in the UK and USA for a long time, but it was only in 1986 that the virus was first isolated. The good news is that, unlike feline enteritis virus, FIV is very fragile and lives for only a short time outside the body. Thus, the risk of indirect (fomite) transmission on hands, food bowls, tools etc. is really very low. Infection is usually by biting, and the risk of infection is greater in cats that go outside and are likely to get into fights. This is the reason why the disease is found in older cats. It is particularly prevalent in feral cats. It appears to have a worldwide prevalence.

Signs: Diagnosis can be difficult. Sometimes the cat has diarrhoea or mild conjunctivitis, with enlarged lymph nodes a few weeks after the original infection. In other cats, there may be no signs for months or even years. The main effect of infection is that the cat's immune system becomes incompetent, hence the name 'immunodeficiency disease'.

Other signs include sneezing, snuffling, raised temperature, diarrhoea and kidney failure. In other words, infection with FIV lays the cat open to all the common feline infections. Ultimately, the cat is so weakened by these that it has to be put to sleep on humane grounds.

Treatment: No routine vaccine is available but spread in multi-cat households can be successfully restricted with the help of your veterinarian. This often involves tests on all resident cats.

In many ways, FIV is similar to HIV in humans. However, HIV cannot infect cats and the owner cannot pick up FIV or develop AIDS from FIV-positive cats.

FELINE LEUKAEMIA VIRUS – FeLV

FeLV is the other major 'resistance lowering virus'. It was discovered in Glasgow in 1964. Like FIV, it is a fragile virus and cannot be transmitted by fomites. It is usually transmitted by direct contact, mostly as a result of licking and grooming, since it is found in the saliva of infected individuals. Kittens under four months of age are very susceptible. After this age, there is a gradual increasing resistance to infection.

FeLV can cross the placenta so that kittens born from an infected queen are likely to be infected. The incubation period from infection with the virus to development of the disease can be from months to years.

Figures show that approximately 85 per cent of infected cats die within 3.5 years of infection. The main effect of infection is to suppress the cat's immune system so that infections like flu, enteritis and FIP are easily picked up.

FeLV can also cause anaemia, leukaemia and lymphosarcoma (a type of cancer). Today effective vaccines are available and are recommended in situations where individual cats are at risk. However, before vaccination your vet may recommend a simple

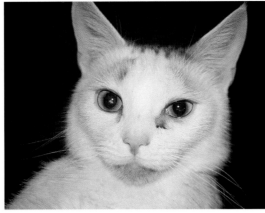

Ocular discharge (left eye) following cat flu.

FeLV test to ensure the cat has not already picked up the virus. *Vaccination will not protect the cat if it is already infected.*

Cat breeders maintain their stock free of FeLV by rigorously ensuring that only cats with FeLV negative certificates come into their catteries. This applies not only to breeding stock but also to any boarders taken in.

FELINE INFECTIOUS ANAEMIA (FIA)

This is caused by an organism known as *Haemobartonella felis* (which belongs to a class of micro-organisms called mycoplasmas). It invades and destroys the erythrocytes or red blood cells. It is thought the disease is transmitted by biting insects, such as fleas. Many cats are infected without becoming anaemic and these are known as silent (or latent) carriers. FIA is stress related. There is also a correlation between FIA with FeLV and FIV infections.

Signs: In affected cats, recurrent episodes of severe anaemia, lethargy and dullness occur. Lifting the cat's lip will often give an indication of the severity of the anaemia, since the gums will appear pale or even white. If you are think you cat is anaemic, see your vet without delay. There are many causes of feline anaemia, and FIA is perhaps one of the least common.

RABIES

No discussion on feline viral infections would be complete without at least the mention of rabies. Although mercifully absent in the UK, it is a problem in many parts of the United States. All mammals, including humans and some birds and bats, are susceptible. The virus is present in the saliva of infected animals and commonly spread by biting. In Europe, the red fox is always considered the most common vector, although this danger has been significantly reduced in parts of northern Europe as a result of widespread of use of vaccines administered via bait to the sylvan fox population. In the US, the raccoon is the main vector.

Mandatory vaccination of dogs and cats is required in many parts of the world including the US. With the advent of the Pets Travel Scheme (PETS) rabies vaccination is now widely available in the UK and is mandatory for any animals entering the UK under PETS.

PART III

COMPLEMENTARY THERAPIES

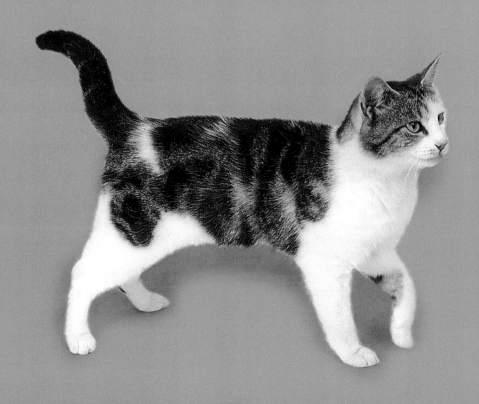

ANOTHER WAY FORWARD

Chapter 20

Complementary and alternative medicine (CAM) is the term used by the conventionally medically trained to cover a variety of approaches to injury and disease, which can be used alongside conventional medicine or, in some cases, instead of the usual medical approach. CAM is really an all-embracing title. Some of the disciplines involved, for example traditional Chinese medicine (TCM), the most well-known component of which is **acupuncture,** are based on practices that have evolved over many thousands of years, thus having a considerably longer history than our Western 'traditional' medicine.

The term CAM, although all-embracing is nevertheless descriptive. It is also useful in that it does not make any attempt to differentiate 'alternative' and 'complementary' treatments.

Complementary medicine covers a variety of approaches to injury and disease that can be used alongside conventional medicine. When these same treatments are used on their own, without any input from conventional medicine, they are referred to as alternative medicine. Many people new to complementary and alternative medicine are unaware that many of the same techniques can be used in either capacity. Homoeopathy, for example, lends itself very well to certain simple first-aid situations, e.g. arnica is especially useful for the treatment of severe bruising. Because of the tremendous dilutions used in homoeopathy, arnica can never do any harm and most cats will accept administration by mouth because the medicine is virtually tasteless.

In consequence, arnica is a useful homoeopathic remedy to use as a first-aid remedy when there has been any trauma involving bleeding or bruising. In this first-aid situation, it is being used as an alternative therapy. It is important that you always explain to your vet what you have given to the cat on subsequent examination. If it is appropriate to continue with the same homoeopathic remedy, in conjunction with conventional treatment dispensed by your veterinary surgeon, the same holistic therapy then becomes complementary therapy. I hope this makes the C and the A in CAM a little clearer.

CAM, as a whole, depends upon two important concepts, irrespective of the type of therapy involved (e.g. homoeopathy, acupuncture etc.). They are:
1. That the medicine used is 'natural'

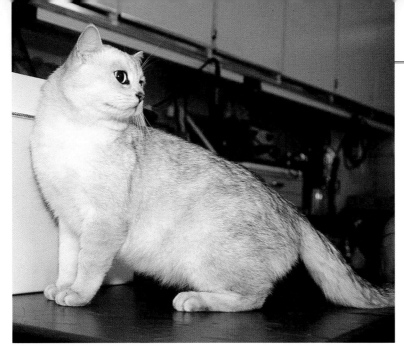

Increasingly, the veterinary profession is ready to accept that alternative therapies have a part to play.

2. That holistic principles are employed in its selection. In other words, it is not just the condition but, importantly, the whole patient that is assessed and then treated.

Thus, holistic means that the patient, no matter whether it be a person or a cat, is considered as a whole rather than being thought of as a collection of various organs or tissues that make up the body, as is the case with conventional medicine.

PROS AND CONS
Perhaps, hardly surprisingly, complementary and alternative medicine can arouse strong feelings. Some conventionalists claim that any CAM is "jiggery pokery," of no use, and can, on some occasions, be dangerous and should never be used. On the other hand, others will maintain that conventional treatment is unnecessary. Their argument is that CAM techniques were used to treat disease long before conventional medicine was established. They believe that conventional (or Western) treatment approaches the disease from the wrong perspective whereas CAM, depending on a holistic approach to the animal, results in the selection of treatments that are natural, will suit the patient and have stood the test of time.

My personal view is that it is likely that the truth lies somewhere between the two extremes. Brought up and trained as a conventionalist as far as my veterinary abilities are concerned, and with the experience of more than half a century of practice, I am very aware of the shortcomings in the conventional approach both to diagnose and treat many common feline conditions.

My work as a forensic veterinary surgeon and expert witness very soon brought me into contact with CAM, about which I was disgracefully ignorant. It soon became clear that if I was to fulfil my role, as far as forensic input was concerned, I had to learn more about CAM. The more I learned, the more I came to respect established holistic techniques – although, in many cases, I did not understand how they worked. However, it was very obvious that in many of the cases I investigated, these techniques either had worked in hastening recovery alongside conventional methods, or had beneficial results used as a last resort following little or no improvement following conventional treatment.

HOLISTIC TREATMENT FOR CATS
The main areas of CAM for cats include **acupuncture, homoeopathy** and **herbal medicine**. Today there also are many other types of 'holistic' treatment, including **aromatherapy, Bach Flower therapy, magneto-therapy** (also known as **bioenergetic therapy**) and, of course, physical therapy, which includes **massage, chiropractic** and **physiotherapy**.

A brief overview of the commonly practised holistic feline therapies follows. Today, there are many veterinary surgeons trained in the use of these and other techniques. If you feel that your cat would benefit from such treatment, discuss it with your vet in the first instance, and ask if a referral can be arranged.

VETERINARY ACUPUNCTURE

Although used in China for over 4,000 years, acupuncture only reached the West in the 1920s, and its use in veterinary medicine commenced about 30 years later. It is now a widely accepted form of treatment, particularly as far as cats are concerned. It is part of traditional Chinese medicine (TCM), which also includes herbal medicine and natural diets. Today, there are an increasing number of conventionally trained veterinary surgeons who are also trained in the use of acupuncture.

Acupuncture is true holistic medicine. From the viewpoint of traditional Chinese medicine (TCM), illness or disease is the result of imbalance of the internal body life force (Qi) often called 'life energy'. Energy patterns both in man and animals follow meridians or channels through the body. In order to flow properly, there must be a balance between Yin and Yang, "the eternal opposites". Yang is considered the positive element and Yin the negative. These are closely interrelated and neither can exist without the other. Disease is said

to occur when the balance of Yin and Yang is upset, resulting in either an excess or a deficiency of one or the other.

Acupuncture is considered to be one of the ways in which this balance is restored. It involves the stimulation of areas on the surface of the body that have direct and intimate relationship with the internal organs through the meridians. With acupuncture, fine needles are inserted in these points, which are situated on the meridians. It is considered that the body produces specific physiological responses that rebalances the life forces and thus cures the patient.

In TCM, acupuncture is not used in isolation but in collaboration with herbal medicine and "dietary wisdom." It is possible that some of the failures with modern veterinary acupuncture are due to lack of full dietary and herbal medicine support, which is part of the original concept.

Acupuncture can be used as alternative therapy (e.g. in the case of lameness due to sprains or strains), and also complementary to traditional methods of treatment, e.g. following major surgery.

VETERINARY HOMOEOPATHY

Homoeopathy, like acupuncture, is an ancient system of medicine. Its popularity in the Western world stems primarily from the work of the German physician, Samuel Hahnemann

(1755-1843). It is based on the principle that like cures like, which he discovered using Peruvian bark (*Cinchona officinalis*) for the successful treatment of malaria. The bark contains quinine and Hahnemann found it could cure a patient with malaria, and yet in the healthy patient Cinchona bark could cause similar signs to malaria.

Hahnemann also discovered that serial dilutions of curative substances, which must include sufficient "**succussion**" (violent agitation) at each stage, were less and less able to produce any harmful effects, yet became more and more powerful as a cure. The combined process of dilution and succession is called **potentization**. The resulting dilutions are termed **potencies**.

Dilutions of 1:100 are designated by the letter C. Thus, arnica 30C is produced by adding one part of arnica to 99 parts of a mixture of water and alcohol. This is then agitated (succussed) to give a potency of 1C. In turn, one part of this solution is added to another 99 parts of the diluent, which results in a potency of 2C, and so on, until arnica 30C is produced.

These dilutions are too great for any of the original substance in the solution to be detected. The theory is that the curative value depends upon the energy stored within the potency. As a result of the repeated dilutions, homoeopathic remedies are very safe.

In most conditions, potencies of between 6C and 30C are suitable, but conditions such as abscesses or some behavioural problems may warrant the use of much higher potencies, e.g. 200C or 1M. This, in Western terms, is an even more dilute solution, but according to homoeopathic theory (because of succussion), more energy laden.

Homoeopathic remedies are available today in the form of pills, which can be crushed for administration, or liquids. It is important not to touch the tablets with bare hands during administration since the potency can be seriously affected.

Paradoxically, it appears not to matter if the whole dose is not administered as long as some of the preparation enters the cat's mouth. Once the signs have improved, medication is usually reduced or stopped.

VETERINARY PHYSIOTHERAPY

Physical therapy in the form of physiotherapy has long been part of feline veterinary treatment for certain conditions, particularly rehabilitation after locomotory problems, such as fractures involving the pelvis and spine. While in practice, I relied heavily upon my human physiotherapy

HERBAL MEDICINE

Most conventionalists are reasonably comfortable with the concept of herbal medicine since it was the true forbearer of modern conventional medicines, many of which originally derived from plants.

However, it should be remembered that the approach in herbal medicine is different. Herbal medicine utilises the natural properties of plants which, when used medicinally, are presented in a less purified and refined form – and in much lower concentrations – than in modern drugs originally derived from plants. Examples of this are salicylic acid (aspirin), derived originally from willow (or meadowsweet), and digitalis, a heart drug that originates from the foxglove, common in country gardens. Even morphine, today still highly valued as a powerful opioid analgesic, derived originally from the opium poppy.

colleagues for advice regarding massage and exercise techniques to act as "support" treatment for many of my feline orthopaedic cases. A few years ago, the Royal Veterinary College, London led the world in instituting a degree in veterinary physiotherapy, so that today specialist veterinary physiotherapists are available to advise on massage and exercise techniques specially designed with the cat's unique anatomy in mind.

This is a good example of where the boundary between conventional treatment and CAM becomes blurred.

Veterinary physiotherapy, in view of its history and universal acceptance within the profession, must surely be considered a conventional technique, whereas chiropractic is considered very definitely part of CAM.

CHIROPRACTIC

Chiropractic is based on the theory that the pressure on the nerves by displaced vertebrae prevent their proper functioning, and lead to disease or non-functioning of the part they serve. The art of chiropractic involves repositioning these bones and relieving this pressure. Thus, to me, perhaps naively, it appears that chiropractic is really a specialised form of physiotherapy. This then leads to the question of the role of osteopathy. This is a system of alternative medicine depending on manipulative techniques to detect and correct faulty structures. I find it convenient to regard chiropractic as 'specialised' osteopathy, dealing only with the spinal vertebrae, whereas osteopathy encompasses the whole skeleton – although I realise this is a very simplistic view.

Many people today find these forms of holistic and/or alternative medicine of benefit for the relief of a variety of

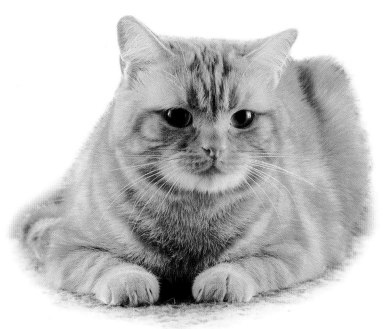

It is always best to consult your veterinary surgeon for an initial diagnosis.

skeletal and other problems, both for themselves and their pets. However, it should be borne in mind that although our pets have a whole range of health problems similar to us, they are in many ways different. Although you may swear by your chiropractor or osteopath for the miraculous results achieved when you "put your back out" and were in agony, remember it is prudent always to consult your veterinary surgeon in the first instance, even if your pet does appear to have similar symptoms. The diagnosis is sometimes entirely different.

That said, do not be afraid to request a referral either to a veterinary osteopath or chiropractor, or to the person with whom you have experience and, importantly, in whom you have faith. With this level of communication you can feel confident you have done the very best for your pet.

PART III

INDEX

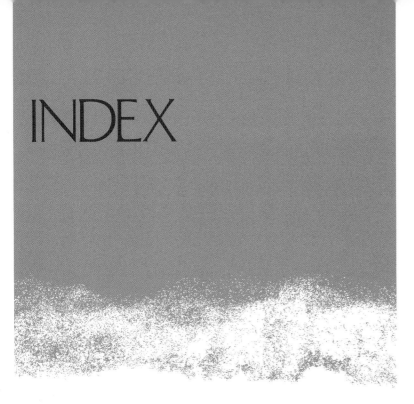